Missionary Women, Leprosy and Indigenous Australians, 1936–1986

"In this clear-sighted, sensitive and deeply researched book, Charmaine Robson provides a compelling account of Indigenous leprosy sufferers and the women missionaries who cared for them in mid-twentieth century Australia. She sheds new light on the politics of public health, the spirituality of care and the different ways in which Indigenous patients made their own lives in sites of incarceration and suffering."

—Anne O'Brien, *Professor of History in the School of Humanities and Languages at University of New South Wales, Australia*

"Packed within Robson's deeply researched account we find several stories: of caring regimes that were severely disciplinary; of Indigenous Australians' terror, adaptation and gratitude; of Catholic Church compassion prodding bewildered and miserly governments. Most of all, Robson illuminates the professionalism of missionary women. Grounded in their faith, they resolved to make a future for people who seemed not to have one. Vividly evoking scenes that were deliberately sequestered, Robson makes these unlikely communities of healing exemplars of settler colonial history's moral burden."

—Tim Rowse, *Emeritus Professor, Institute for Culture and Society, Western Sydney University, Australia*

Charmaine Robson

Missionary Women, Leprosy and Indigenous Australians, 1936–1986

palgrave
macmillan

Charmaine Robson
School of Humanities and Languages
University of New South Wales
Sydney, NSW, Australia

ISBN 978-3-031-05795-3 ISBN 978-3-031-05796-0 (eBook)
https://doi.org/10.1007/978-3-031-05796-0

This Palgrave Macmillan imprint is published by the registered company Springer Nature Switzerland AG
The registered company address is: Gewerbestrasse 11, 6330 Cham, Switzerland

Acknowledgements

This project started life in the old School of History at the University of New South Wales, so my first thanks go to the people there who were so important to its realisation. Anne O'Brien, as my doctoral supervisor was, and remains, a source of constant encouragement, brilliant ideas, and unending patience. Thanks go also to my co-supervisor, Grace Karskens, for her inspiration, enthusiasm, and support at all times. I am grateful for receiving an Australian Postgraduate Award scholarship, and for the continued support of UNSW through my adjunct lectureship position.

Following the footsteps of the religious women and men in this book took me around Australia, and I am appreciative of the many people who welcomed me into their private worlds and precious archives to share their information. Special thanks go to Sr. Patricia Rhatigan and Helen Mary Martin of the Sisters of St John of God Heritage Centre in Broome, Western Australia, and to Helen Lucas of the Townsville Cathedral Archives, and the late Bishop Michael Putney, for their trust and invaluable assistance. Thanks also go to the Missionaries of the Sacred Heart and the Daughters of Our Lady of the Sacred Heart, both in Kensington, Sydney, for access to their archives and for copying and scanning images, especially to Sr. Evelyn Page and the late Sr. Shirley Bates. I am grateful to archivists Sr Madonna Purcell of the Franciscan Missionaries of Mary in Sydney and Dr. Roberta Cowan of the Pallottine Fathers in Rossmoyne, Western Australia.

To the staff of the UNSW Library, the National Archives of Australia in Canberra and Darwin, the Queensland State Archives, James Cook University, the State Records Office of Western Australia, and the Battye Library, thank-you for your assistance with the primary research intrinsic to this book. To Janie Mason of the Charles Darwin University Nursing Museum, Saadia Thomson Dwyer of the Queensland State Archives, Bronwyn McBurnie of James Cook University, and Fiona Caratozzolo of the State Library of Western Australia, I thank you for your assistance with images. And also, a thank you to Lorraine Bottrell for permission to use the wonderful photographs taken by Stuart Gore.

My deep gratitude goes to the interview participants who warmly shared their memories, allowing such rich and personal insights into this history. In particular, I am appreciative to the anonymous "John," a former leprosarium patient, who gave me so much of his time and confidence. My research gained from his tendency to "talk under wet cement," as he put it. Thanks goes to the many former patients and their families who have helped bring Indigenous people's perspectives to this history by the telling or writing of memories. It is not an easy past to go over. Special thanks are also due to the late Dr. John Hargrave for his hospitality and patience with answering endless questions. Thanks to Melanie Robson for technical assistance and the indexing.

Finally, I am indebted to my family, William, Amelia, and Melanie, for their epic endurance and unstinting support.

Contents

List of Figures

CHAPTER 1

Introduction

Dotted around Australia's vast perimeter lie the physical vestiges of nineteenth and twentieth-century leprosy isolation practices, forlorn islands and verges, too bleak or far-flung for all but forced human habitation. Yielding back to the elements, most divulge little trace of their colonised past; in a few, the baked dirt, pricked with the crosses of human transience, remembers death—but of life, is mute. Four of these sites are linked to a recent and specific phase in Australian public health policy and female missionary endeavour. Between 1931 and 1940, government leprosaria for Indigenous Australians were opened in northern Australia: Channel Island, Northern Territory; Derby, Western Australia; and Fantome Island Queensland. A fourth one, on the Northern Territory coast at East Arm, replaced Channel Island in 1955. Until 1986, when, Derby, the last leprosarium closed, at least 2000 people were removed to these institutions under strict detention laws. Many died while inmates. Others remained for various periods, up to decades, before advances in medicine and policy changes finally permitted their release (Fig. 1.1).

A little-known aspect of these institutions was the participation of Catholic religious Sisters, appointed by respective governments to nurse the patients. Over the approximate fifty years in which they occupied these positions, their duties diversified into administration, patient education, and ancillary health services such as pharmacy, physiotherapy, medical

C. Robson, *Missionary Women, Leprosy and Indigenous Australians, 1936–1986*, https://doi.org/10.1007/978-3-031-05796-0_1

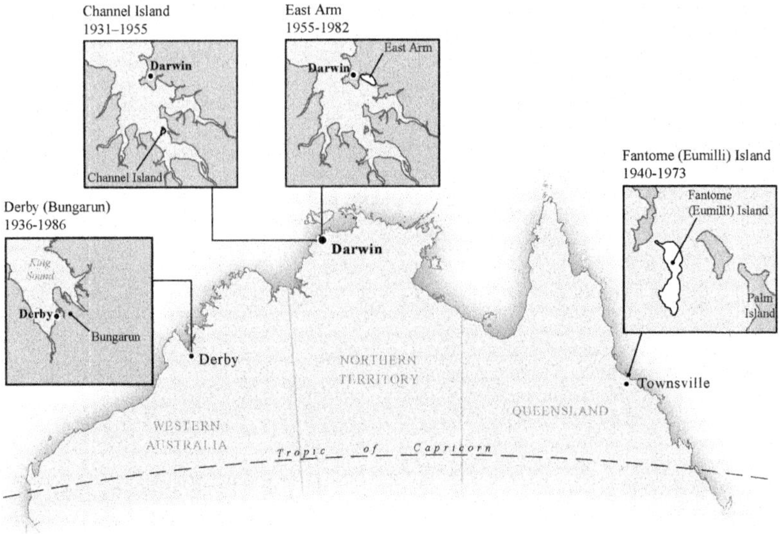

Fig. 1.1 Map of northern Australia showing leprosarium locations (Alan Laver)

research and dentistry, and the training of Indigenous health assistants. Senior Sisters assumed authority over patient discipline and welfare. As nurses, the women implemented public health policy and medical treatment protocols, services for which governments paid their religious communities. As missionary women, they were purveyors of the culture and spirit of their congregations, their individual vocational aspirations, and the expanding missionary ambitions of the Catholic Church. This book investigates how Catholic Sisters, charged with effecting these sometimes conflicting, sometimes intersecting social, religious, and therapeutic ideals, shaped conditions and experiences for Indigenous leprosy-affected people in the twentieth century. It looks, too, at the ways patients managed and responded to institutional life, and their relationships with each other and the Sisters. These missionaries have received little scholarly attention. They have figured in histories that include some discussion of the leprosaria but not with the analysis they warrant.[1] From these studies, little can be learnt of their backgrounds, training, and motivations, all of which critically informed their leprosarium work. The role of the Catholic Church and a new female-centred missionary initiative have been overlooked yet were crucial to the Sisters' entry into the leprosarium apostolate and the continued authority by Catholic male religious over patients' lives.

To date, a full account of leprosy and Australian Indigenous people has not been undertaken, despite the significance of this chapter of history for our understandings of race relations. The forcible removal of people to distant institutions has left in its wake a long shadow across Indigenous communities of northern Australia reminiscent of the Stolen Generations history. The loss and sense of injustice suffered by families and communities when loved ones were removed has not been forgotten. For some communities and individuals, this history has tainted European medical practices, impeding the delivery of badly needed health services to Indigenous people. A collective disquiet about what went on in the leprosaria, and why, continues to haunt some descendants and kinsfolk. They have seen or heard about the painful moments of babies taken from their parents' arms, children whisked from the schoolroom in shame, and men shackled in chains for the march into isolation. They know about the waiting and the longing over the years, and, so often, the bad news, or no news at all. Of the people who did return home, many were in worse shape than when they left. Claims for European medical know-how rang hollow—the constant injections and concoctions that didn't work, or made one violently ill, or came too late for patients to see or walk again. As families understand it, this was not 'treatment,' the description used by Western medicine at the time; it was experimentation. Some assert that people who did not actually have leprosy were taken to the leprosaria. Not surprisingly, these institutions became highly feared and to be avoided at all costs. When effective therapies and shorter inpatient stays were possible from the 1960s, the association of the leprosaria with the fragmentation of families, death and pain remained, despite efforts to lift their image and encourage sufferers to come forward for treatment.[2]

This book seeks to deepen an understanding of Australian missionary work with Indigenous people, within the setting of infectious disease management. It argues that religion played a pivotal role in the implementation of leprosy policy over the years covered by this study, because of the significant involvement of Catholic missionary women, and, to a lesser extent, missionary men. The study draws from recent histories by Katharine Massam and Regina Ganter which stress the Christian spirituality that motivated and directed the work and lives of Catholic and Protestant missionaries.[3] If, as Ganter maintains, "faith needs, after all, to be taken seriously if we wish to understand what powered the mission movement," then it also should be heeded to understand the missionary impulse operating within the leprosaria.[4] Catholic mission histories, especially those with focus on women religious, offer useful comparisons and context. The themes of cultural assimilation, evangelisation, labour, the separation and creation of Indigenous families, Indigenous peoples' agency and resistance, the gendered power dynamics of the Church, and the effect of changing government policy run through works by Christine Choo and Massam with varying emphasis.[5] These themes, although inflected differently where patients were detainees in government public health institutions, also characterised the structures of care in the leprosaria.

Leprosy policy for Indigenous people throughout Australia differed markedly to that for the non-Indigenous, but the extent and nature of the differences have not been fully explored. By illuminating and analysing these differences, this book offers fresh insights to the governance of Indigenous people in a health institution setting. Differential policies easily elude our notice. They cannot be found in public health laws demanding the mandatory removal and detention of leprosy sufferers, as race was not mentioned. But they were apparent in recommendations, decisions, and practices, the most vivid examples of which were the stringent, long-term—sometimes permanent—isolation imposed on Indigenous patients and the creation of separate Indigenous leprosaria. The institutional conditions and systems also varied from those for European patients, including the staffing which for the latter, consisted of lay workers.

The ways race informed government responses to the Australian leprosy epidemic of the twentieth century resounds in the COVID-19 pandemic. In Sydney in 2021, evening curfews, police patrols and military surveillance, and permits for leaving one's home area were introduced in suburbs of socio-economic disadvantage and with high concentrations of migrant and Indigenous communities. The New South Wales Premier denied these measures were racist, but merely addressing areas with high case numbers. The Deputy Police Commissioner suggested otherwise when he stated that residents needed "to understand their responsibilities… especially in south-west Sydney, where there might be some barriers to what people can and cannot do, we would really ask family and friends to explain it to those people what's required of them."[6] Poor compliance here was put down to a kind of ignorance, attributed squarely to non-Anglo-Celtic people, with the implication that their cultures are inimical to responsible hygienic behaviour, when, in fact, structural factors such as types of employment and household sizes rendered these communities vulnerable to infection. Leprosy removals by police or patrol officers, were also based on the notion that Indigenous people's habits and culture were conducive to the spread of disease, even if authorities acknowledged the parts played by substandard living conditions and a lack of health services. This heavy-handed racial targeting in epidemics has a long genealogy in settler nations, perhaps because the panic of public health emergencies brings to the surface the ever-present anxiety about the unassimilated.

This book brings to light the many ways patients made their own lives. Amid the death, illness, oppression, austerity, and separation that characterised the leprosarium, it is easy to overlook the patients' agency in this story. Testimonies by former patients of Australian leprosaria remind us of their resilience rather than their victimisation. They stress friendships and romances, shared experiences, and mutual support between patients, and between patients and Sisters. Munanjahli and South Sea Islander academic, Chelsea Watego, explains: "you will find mob who talk fondly of the mission days not because they believe necessarily that missions or reserves were the solution but that, even in the most oppressive conditions, our mob exercised agency in these places, finding meaning in hardship, never relinquishing our humanity or our humour."[7] The formation of communities and relationships in isolation was integral to these coping mechanisms and, as scholars of leprosy history, Vicki Luker and Jane Buckingham, suggest, exploring them helps to elucidate subjective experiences.[8] But it is important also to recognise the ongoing struggle by patients to keep connections with their home communities as they had not all given up hope of leaving isolation.

The Sisters' approach to patient care was holistic. As well as their nursing duties, they incorporated activities to address minds, bodies, and souls such as music, education, Christian worship, art and crafts, and sports. Simultaneously, they imposed discipline through encouragement of a work ethic, hygienic behaviour, and sexual morality. Their delivery of Western cultural forms and ethos to Indigenous leprosarium populations sought to create stoic 'civilised' societies within the institutions. Warwick Anderson's history of the Culion leprosarium in early twentieth-century Philippines offers some resonances. Far from being of no interest to American authorities, the "colonial leper" was captive to relentless training by staff in the "American ideals of civic responsibility."[9] These lessons could never be truly exercised, however, while patients remained in isolation. It was the same for Indigenous Australian patients, who even after the 1950s when discharge was more likely, remained caught up in a web of structural and legislative restrictions that impeded their independence.

Watura Kusaka's investigation of Culion, however, suggests caution when interpreting the institutional reform of patients or the regulation of their lives. She found that power was limited by patients' own agency, and that they "undermined the colonial order" by absconding, gambling, and refusing to work.[10] In the Australian institutions, these forms of resistance also occurred. Some patients, by refusing to submit to rules and conditions, forced changes to policies. Many challenged the Western cultural models promoted by maintaining traditions and languages, even exchanging them with others. The Sisters, and sometimes doctors, often accommodated or pushed for these kinds of changes to keep patients contented. The patients therefore did hold some power. Highly constrained, it nonetheless gave them some control over their lives and their relationships with other patients.

This book examines another important and much neglected aspect of the history: the role of the wider Catholic Church and individual male missionaries. It argues that by the early 1940s, with Catholic personnel installed in all Indigenous leprosaria and continued authority by local bishops, these institutions had become joint projects of Church and government. As with the northern Christian missions opening in the same period, the leprosaria resonate with what historian Anne O'Brien has called an "intimacy" of relations between "the state and voluntarism" in Australia.[11]

But if, in an era of intense religious sectarianism, the Catholic Church could triumphantly claim the souls of all Australia's Indigenous leprosy patients through this partnership—and, indeed, call the leprosaria 'Catholic missions,'—what was the advantage for the state? Why appoint and maintain Catholic Sisters as senior leprosarium staff for five decades? Why share authority with bishops and priests? These questions are important because they raise the issue of government objectives for the patients. Current historiography argues that the state was indifferent to their welfare, as the predominant aim of the leprosarium was segregation, not care.[12] But governments did take an interest in the patients' lives, if not always with benevolence. Employing qualified Sisters, rather than leaving the patients to their own resources, was one indication. That the women came cheaply or were the only nurses willing to work in a leprosarium was true only to a limited extent as will be explained in a later chapter. By the 1930s, Catholic Sister nurses generally had gained a reputation for clinical professionalism and moral authority, sealed in Catholic hospitals and overseas missions, and doctors and health bureaucrats expected that they would bring these qualities and their nurse training and experience to the leprosaria. The Sisters remained because these expectations were mostly fulfilled, and sometimes exceeded. They were valued assets to governments, even when their views did not align. So the Sisters' work provides a window through which we can understand bureaucratic goals for patients, beyond their removal from society.

* * *

Why was the imperative to keep Indigenous people confined so strong? Leprosy policies directed towards socially subordinated races have been common in colonised societies over different historical periods. A recent study has argued that in eighteenth-century Suriname, Dutch colonists introduced the compulsory segregation of people of African descent to protect white labour.[13] To justify their actions, they constructed racial stereotypes of Africans as morally and physically degenerate, and prone to spreading disease. Although far away in time and place, these findings echo with the Australian experience of leprosy for Indigenous people. Interwar northern Australia, still very much a frontier, brought white male labourers in contact with Indigenous people and diseases imported by migrant workers, prompting a major public health response. Protection of European health to enable their settlement was the issue here. Yet, it was ideas about how Indigenous people lived and behaved that, on entering medical discourse, doomed them to the strictest isolation measures. Racial preconceptions of Indigenous people as irresponsible in matters of hygiene, sex, mobility, and physical intimacy held fast over the ensuing decades, and rationalised continued institutional control, regardless of therapies that reduced infectivity. The policy reflected the more widespread sets of controls imposed by Australian authorities on Indigenous people which were never lightly dispensed with.

The leprosy epidemics in Australia and responses by state and church should be understood in global terms, as scholar Mark Harrison suggests for medical histories.[14] Epidemics did not arise in vacuums but resulted from momentous historical changes. The arrival of leprosy in Australia with successive waves of imported labour after the middle of the nineteenth century was part of the larger-scale transmission of the disease begun centuries earlier through worker migration to the New World. These diasporas followed European settlement and colonisation, and brought leprosy to previously unexposed populations, with devastating results. Similarly, local measures to deal with leprosy responded to international events, biomedical discoveries, and the influence of global humanitarian and health agencies. The exile of the leprosy sufferer from society, whether to islands, asylums, or beyond the limits of the city seems to have transcended cultural, geographical, and temporal boundaries, and could be said to be truly global. However, many historians specifically situate these practices in ancient Judaeo-Christian traditions as found in the Bible.[15] Others point to long-held local conventions of leprosy exclusion and stigma, as in China, and, though not as extreme as in the West, India.[16]

Studies by scholars Zachary Gussow and George S. Tracy, taking the former view, have identified another large movement that affected leprosy policy. They refer to the thousands of Protestant and Catholic missionaries who left Europe from the late nineteenth to the early twentieth century to evangelise non-Christians around the world. They argue that these missionaries "discovered" modern leprosy sufferers and reconceptualised them as the biblical leper, a figure of spiritual and physical affliction.[17] Leprosy sufferers were set apart as missionaries saw them "as a very special group of people," and desired to heal their "disease of the soul."[18] Yet, these and subsequent supporting studies offer few insights about the practical care given by Christian missionaries, and therefore the full impact of this international missionary imperative remains unknown.[19]

Internationally, of the studies that allude to the care or oversight of leprosy patients by Catholic and other missionaries, few have drawn findings from the voices and documented actions of Catholic Sister nurses. These histories either do not analyse the women's healthcare work or confine it to a narrow period, generally the late nineteenth to early twentieth century.[20] This leaves a significant gap in the historiography, considering that by 1951, Catholic women religious were nursing approximately 72,000 patients at 220 leprosaria around the world.[21] As historian Barbra Mann Wall has noted, histories have often relied on religious discourse to represent the work of medical missionaries and their attitudes towards their patients.[22] Histories of leprosy care in particular have relied on biblical extracts, ministers' sermons and religious magazines as sources.[23] Their influence cannot be dismissed, but they cannot reveal "the lived reality of mission work on the ground where health care actually took place," to quote Mann Wall.[24] The historical silence around women religious in the leprosaria is, in Hilary Carey's words, part of a broader "tendency of nuns…to remain veiled in historical narratives."[25] Sioban Nelson's point that Catholic Sisters in the nineteenth century avoided publicity and renounced their individual identities held true until the 1960s when restrictions were eased under Vatican II.[26]

The work of the leprosarium Sisters features in celebratory histories of Catholic women's congregations and Indigenous missions written from inside the Church or Catholic orders. They depict the women as committed individuals who withstood the many challenges of the work—impoverishment, lack of food, the proximity of war, and harsh tropical environments—strengthened by their faith and determination.[27] These texts position the leprosarium Sisters as rescuers of Indigenous leprosy sufferers who are represented as the victims of uncaring white Australians, and their own primitive helplessness.[28] However, portrayals of 'abandoned' patients mask the love and support their relatives and communities had for them, and the fact that they were only under missionaries' care because they had no choice. This study takes a critical approach to the Sisters' work and seeks, as Watego warns white writers, to avoid its glorification "in a very real story of everyday and ongoing colonial violence."[29]

Scope

This book spans the time frame in which Catholic Sisters staffed the leprosaria, 1937 to 1986, coinciding with the period in which separate leprosaria for Indigenous people operated, except for Channel Island which opened in 1931 with lay staff. Four women's religious communities served at the institutions. The Sisters of St John of God, based in Western Australia's Kimberley district, took up their positions at Derby shortly after it opened in 1937. Their offshoot community, the Sisters of Our Lady Help of Christians arrived to work at Fantome Island in 1940, and was replaced with the international order, the Franciscan Missionaries of Mary five years later. In 1943, amid the bombing of Darwin by the Japanese, the Daughters of Our Lady of the Sacred Heart took up the nursing at nearby Channel Island, and continued when the leprosarium moved to the mainland at East Arm. Following the installation of these nurses, their congregations sent more Sisters to serve in various roles such as school-teaching, cooking, and housekeeping. The Catholic Church had yet another presence in these institutions. Religious Brothers were engaged as superintendents at Channel Island and priests were resident or semi-resident chaplains at all leprosaria.

This study straddles two eras in world leprosy epidemiology history: the periods prior to, and after, the discovery of effective drug therapy. Before the 1940s, leprosy was treated cheaply and simply with the extract of a natural oil, and although clinicians made great claims for its efficacy, it was not until the sulphone class of drugs was introduced that noteworthy improvements took place. Worldwide, patients were found to be no longer infectious, their symptoms cleared up, and many were discharged from leprosy villages and institutions. It would be overstating the success of this treatment to claim that everyone responded well, but, overall, this period marked a triumphant turning point for disease control and for the fate of many sufferers.

There was little these new drugs could do for another category of leprosarium inpatient. These people had already acquired one or more of the many debilitating effects of the disease, such as blindness, deformities caused by the destruction of peripheral nerves, and paralysis, before modern drug treatment had been available to forestall their onset.[30] In accordance with earlier procedures for badly affected limbs, they might have had one or more amputations. Usually no longer infectious, some of these long-term sufferers were known as 'burnt-out cases.' Their residence in a leprosarium had more to do with their support, rather than their confinement. Surgical and physiotherapeutic advances made available to varying extents from the 1950s helped some of these people regain their independence but for many, while the leprosarium remained open, it was where they would spend the rest of their days.

Methodology

A diverse selection of primary sources was consulted for the research in this book, including missionary and government archival records; contemporary medical journals, books and reports; newspapers and books containing memories by former patients and their communities; and oral interviews. Annual reports of health and Indigenous affairs departments trace patient statistics, therapeutic developments, and other changes in the leprosaria. Papal documents, Catholic conference proceedings and periodicals were valuable for understanding the church and missionary attitudes and policies. Correspondence within and between different departments, and between government and the Sisters, bishops and priests, have been extremely fruitful for the revelation not only of policy and practice, but of objectives, ideas, conflict, and concerns. Letters between missionaries and their religious superiors are informative about the spiritual purpose of missionary work.

The author conducted interviews with several Sisters from Channel Island, East Arm and Derby leprosaria. Interviews with other Sisters were available in state libraries. The oral interview retrieved information unavailable in other sources and also helped to elucidate meanings of the leprosarium experience for the Sisters. The oral interview can retrieve perspectives of "ordinary people," those whose class, race, and gender, for example, limit opportunities for their voices to be heard.[31] As Carole Garibaldi Rogers argues for Catholic Sisters, it helps to expose the role of women religious in the public arena and their negotiation of gender constraints imposed by the Catholic patriarchy.[32] Nevertheless, the women interviewed maintained a reserve about their achievements and tended to deflect conversation to those of others, such as the patients and doctors. Another limitation to the interviews was the intrusion of intervening experiences in shaping memory. Portelli's comment that "acts considered legitimate and even normal or necessary in the past may be now literally cast out of the tradition" applied to some Sisters who espoused views that seemed dissonant with some of the attitudes evident in contemporaneous documents.[33] They had all begun their leprosarium work before the impact of Vatican II, and had since come to terms with issues such as ecumenism and Indigenous self-determination.

The voices of Indigenous people in regard to their experiences of leprosy policy are widely scattered fragments in archival correspondence, edited books, newspapers, and interviews. Oral interviews with former patients including one with the author, were informative of personal perspectives and leprosaria conditions. Most are memories recounted years after the leprosarium experience, but a few come directly from the past, for example, petitions and letters of complaint to governments. Much can also be learnt about the patients in correspondence by authorities, if read with caution—not only the conditions they lived under, but some of their responses. Photographs can be very helpful historical sources but in this book, only images in which patients cannot be clearly identified have been used, in consideration for the privacy of the subjects and their families.

Context

Leprosy is a mildly infectious bacterial disease which affects mainly the skin and nerves. In its less invasive form, known as 'tuberculoid,' the bacteria remain confined to skin lesions and peripheral nerves. It can progress to the more contagious 'lepromatous' form where the bacteria spreads through the body, causing a range of serious systemic illnesses, leading sometimes to death. In most people, the disease lies somewhere between these two extremes.[34] Advances in therapy have been slow, partly because in vitro cultivation of the bacteria has not been possible and the exact means of person-to-person transmission remains unknown.[35] What is known, and has been known since the interwar years, is that leprosy is not easily transmitted but probably occurs through droplet or skin contact. Because leprosy has a very long incubation period, sometimes as long as twenty years, diagnosis may not be possible until the disease has been spread to others, and therefore the effectiveness of isolation as a measure of control has been debated.

Leprosy was almost certainly unknown in Indigenous Australians before the late nineteenth century, but from the late 1920s, when cases among them began to outnumber all others, they became the focus of rigid government policies, including strict isolation in the leprosarium. The removals of Indigenous people can be situated in the context of segregative public health practices in the colonies of Western imperial powers from the late nineteenth century. Indigenous inhabitants or non-white migrants, especially Indians and Chinese, were often the targets of state responses to leprosy and other disease outbreaks, reflecting the colonial hegemony and medicalised constructions of non-European races as intrinsically susceptible to disease and dangerously contagious.[36] In Western Australia and Queensland, Indigenous people diagnosed with sexually transmitted diseases were removed to island lock hospitals.[37]

The governing of Indigenous Australians has, itself, a tradition of segregation. The protection acts introduced across Australia from the late nineteenth to the early twentieth century were the main mechanisms for removing Indigenous people to government reserves and missions. Created purportedly to safeguard the race from exploitation, venereal diseases and other presumed ill-effects of their association with Europeans and Asians and based on the assumption that the race would eventually die out, the legislation empowered governments to control Indigenous people's movements, their reproduction, and their labour.[38] The acts also allowed for the removal of Indigenous children to missions and government homes. Removal and confinement under leprosy control measures were thus "problematically familiar," as historian Alison Bashford has pointed out.[39]

'Protection' operated in parallel with the White Australia Policy, to privilege the prosperity, health, and personal liberty of the white Australian, while excising the non-white, spatially and from civil rights. The north, with its racially diverse populations and proximity to southeast Asia, undermined the notion of the Anglo-Australian national identity. Coastal towns such as Broome and Darwin were home to families of mixed Asian, Indigenous, and European descent, and non-white residents worked the local industries such as pearling and mining. The protection laws aimed to prevent further interracial contact, although they were modified at local level for Indigenous workers whose labour was essential.[40] Policymakers sought particularly to prevent sexual relations between white men and Indigenous women, believing them responsible for enfeebling the white race through the spread of diseases such as leprosy and syphilis and the birth of mixed-race children. This aim became more pressing with the influx of white males in the push to develop these regions over the first half of the twentieth century, and amendments to the protection acts in the 1930s brought new stringency. Protection of the white race from the people and from the inhospitable environment of the north became the subject of biomedical and anthropological thought. It informed practitioners of tropical medicine in Australia, the same doctors who were to influence leprosy policies, designate treatments for leprosy patients and, in many cases, personally attend them.

In the 1950s, Australian governments changed their policy approach from one of protection to assimilation, recognising that Indigenous people were not going to die out and that a future for them in society was to be carved out. Many, however, found the controls over their lives increased. They came under greater bureaucratic scrutiny as access to the promised equality with whites was conditional on their adoption of idealised European ways of living and working, and, in some cases, on their good health. Yet, the assimilation policy, coinciding with medical breakthroughs in leprosy treatments, ultimately benefitted leprosy patients in the Northern Territory, where health reform was most strongly tied to Indigenous policy.

Chapters

Chapter 2 provides the deep historical framework for the system that ultimately defined twentieth-century leprosy policy for Indigenous Australians. It explains the religious and cultural significance of leprosy for Western Christian societies and briefly traces societal responses to this disease by professed Christian men and women since ancient times. It briefly examines Christian missions in Australia and links modern Australian Catholic religious to their nineteenth-century Irish and Continental foundations and the concomitant Christian missionary outreach to the Australian colonies. A brief history of leprosy in Australia in the period up to 1924 is provided.

Chapter 3 opens in 1925 to examine the social and medical forces that shaped government decisions to pursue stringent leprosy policies for Indigenous people, including the establishment of leprosaria at Channel Island (1931), Derby (1936), and Fantome Island (1940). Chapter 4 explains the factors that led to the appointments of the nursing Sisters at these institutions, and includes the histories of the Catholic women's congregations and the growth of an interwar Catholic missionary outreach in northern Australia. Chapters 5–7 examine the leprosarium work of the Sisters in detail over the years 1937 to 1955. They introduce the patients and other staff members, and explain institutional conditions. They consider separately the themes of nursing and medical care; the incorporation of education, labour, and cultural pursuits; and patient discipline and protest, sexual morality and reproduction. Chapter 8 examines the part played by male missionaries in the leprosaria, focusing first on their conceptualisation of the leprosarium as a Catholic mission and their roles as chaplains and government superintendents, and, second, the meaning of the leprosy apostolate to individual Brothers and priests.

Chapter 9 begins in 1955 and traces the impact of post-war advances in medical science and new Indigenous welfare policies on Australian Indigenous patients, and on the positions of the Sister nurses, with a strong focus on the Northern Territory, where a new mainland leprosarium at East Arm replaced Channel Island. Chapter 10 explains the continued constraints on the rights of Indigenous patients through this later period, despite some gains in health and welfare. It discusses ways in which some staff worked or fought to have the therapeutic and social benefits of this more modern period delivered to Indigenous patients. Chapter 11, the final chapter, documents the closing of the institutions in the 1970s and 1980s, and discusses consequences of leprosarium life for Indigenous people after their discharge, using their own voices. Ex-patients' memories are also used to bring out their own perspective of this history. This chapter closes with the book's conclusion.

Notes

1. Saunders, Suzanne. 1986. "A Suitable Island Site": Leprosy in the Northern Territory and the Channel Island Leprosarium 1880–1955. B.A. Hons. Diss. Murdoch University; Maguire, John. 1991. 'The Fantome Island Leprosarium.' In *Health and Healing in Tropical Australia and Papua New Guinea*, ed. Roy Macleod and Donald Denoon. Townsville: James Cook University Press, 142–148; Carey, Hilary M. 1998. 'Subordination, Invisibility and Chosen Work: Missionary Nuns and Australian Aborigines c.1900–1949.' *Australian Feminist Studies* 13 (28), 251–267; Briscoe, Gordon. 2003. *Counting, Health and Identity: A History of Aboriginal Health and Demography in Western Australia and Queensland 1900–1940*. Canberra: Aboriginal Studies Press; Robson, Charmaine. 2007. On Fantome Island: A History of Indigenous Exile and Community. B.A. Hons. Diss. University of New South Wales; Genever, Geoffrey. 2008. 'Queensland's Black Leper Colony.' *Queensland Review* 15 (2), 59–68; Parsons, Meg. 2008. Spaces of Disease: the Creation and Management of Aboriginal Health and Disease in Queensland, 1900–1970. Ph.D diss. University of Sydney.
2. Hunter, Ernest. 1991. 'Stains on the Caring Mantle: Doctors in Aboriginal Australia have a history.' *Medical Journal of Australia* 155 (11–12), 779–783; Robson, Charmaine. 2018. 'Medical Experimentation and Indigenous Intergenerational Memory in the Context of Twentieth-Century Hansen's Disease Treatment in Australia.' *Health and History* 20 (2), 54–74.
3. Massam, Katharine. 2020. *A Bridge Between: Spanish Benedictine Missionary Women in Australia*. Australian Capital Territory: ANU Press; Ganter, Regina. 2018. *The Contest for Aboriginal Souls: European Missionary Agendas in Australia*. Australian Capital Territory: ANU Press.
4. Ganter, *The Contest for Aboriginal Souls*, 169.
5. Choo, Christine. 2001. *Mission Girls: Aboriginal Women on Catholic Missions in the Kimberley, Western Australia, 1900–1950*. Crawley: University of Western Australia Press.

6. Livingston, Tom. 2021. '"This is not about Discrimination, Not About Racism": NSW Police Patrol South-West Sydney.' July 9. Nine News Online.
   https://www.9news.com.au/national/coronavirus-sydney-update-extra-police-patrolling-south-west-lgas-lockdown-breaches-cases-surge/676bd916-6f0d-4d52-957b-0dc3ed2b1f90 Accessed 29 Jan 2022.
7. Watego, Chelsea. 2021. *Another Day in the Colony*. St. Lucia: University of Queensland Press, 60.
8. Luker, Vicki and Jane Buckingham. 2017. 'Histories of Leprosy: Subjectivities, Community and Pacific Worlds.' *Journal of Pacific History* 52 (3), 267.
9. Anderson, Warwick. 1998. 'Leprosy and Citizenship.' *Positions* 6 (3), 723.
10. Kusaka, Wataru. 2017. 'Discipline and desire: Hansen's Disease patients reclaim life in Culion, 1900–1930s.' *Social Science Diliman*. 13 (2), 19.
11. O'Brien, Anne. 2015. *Philanthropy and Settler Colonialism*. Basingstoke: Palgrave Macmillan, 5.
12. Saunders, Suzanne. 1990. 'Isolation: The Development of Leprosy Prophylaxis in Australia.' *Aboriginal History* 14, 175; Bashford, Alison. 2004. *Imperial Hygiene: A Critical History of Colonialism, Nationalism and Public Health*. Sydney: Palgrave, 100–101.
13. Snelders, Stephen, Leo van Bergen and Frank Huisman. 2019. 'Leprosy and the Colonial Gaze: Comparing the Dutch West and East Indies, 1750–1950.' *Social History of Medicine* 34 (2), 617–618. See also Kakar, Sanjiv. 1996. 'Leprosy in British India, 1860–1940: Colonial Politics and Missionary Medicine.' *Medical History*, 221; Gussow, Zachary. 1989. *Leprosy, Racism & Public Health: Social Policy in Chronic Disease Control*. Boulder: Westview Press, 102; Mawani, R. 2003.'"The Island of the Unclean:" Race, Colonialism and "Chinese Leprosy" in British Columbia, 1891–1924.' *Law, Social Justice & Global Development Journal* 1, http://elj.warwick.ac.uk/global/03-1/mawani.html, 13; Obregon, Diana. 2002. 'Building National Medicine: Leprosy and Power in Colombia, 1870–1910.' *Social History of Medicine* 15 (1), 108.
14. Harrison, Mark. 2015. 'A Global Perspective: Reframing the History of Health, Medicine, and Disease.' *Bulletin of the History of Medicine* 89 (4), 653, 661.
15. Watts, Sheldon. 1997. *Epidemics and History: Disease, Power and Imperialism*. New Haven & London: Yale University Press, 41; Joseph, D. George. 2003. 'Essentially Christian, Eminently Philanthropic: The Mission to Lepers in British India.' *Historia Ciencias Saude—Manguinhos Rio de Janeiro* 10 (supplement 1), 249; Moran, Michelle T. 2007. *Colonizing Leprosy: Imperialism and the Politics of Public Health in the United States*. Chapel Hill: University of North. Carolina Press, 6. See also Saunders, 'A Suitable Island Site' (1989), 1–2.

16. Leung, Angela Ki Che. 2009. *Leprosy in China*. New York: Columbia University Press, 4–6; Buckingham, Jane. 2002. *Leprosy in Colonial India*. Basingstoke: Palgrave, 31–35.
17. Gussow, Zachary and George S. Tracy. 1970. 'Stigma and the Leprosy Phenomenon: The Social History of a Disease in the Nineteenth and Twentieth Centuries.' *Bulletin of the History of Medicine* 44:5, 446.
18. Gussow, Zachary. 1989. *Leprosy, Racism & Public Health: Social Policy in Chronic Disease Control*. Boulder: Westview Press, 210–211.
19. Smith Kipp, Rita. 1994. 'The Evangelical Uses of Leprosy.' *Social Science and Medicine* 39 (2), 167–168; Bernabeu-Mestre, Josep and Teresa Ballester-Artigues. 2004. 'Disease as a Metaphorical Resource: The Fontilles Philanthropic Initiative in the Fight Against Leprosy 1901–1932.' *Social History of Medicine* 17 (3), 416–417; Moran, *Colonizing Leprosy*, 5, 81; Worboys, Michael. 2000. 'The Colonial World as Mission and Mandate: Leprosy and Empire 1900–1940.' *Osiris* 15, 209, 214; Vaughan, Megan. 1991. *Curing Their Ills: Colonial Power & African Illness*. Stanford: Stanford University Press, 84; Watts, *Epidemics and History*, 43, 83; Joseph, 'Essentially Christian', 249; Kakar, Sanjiv. 1996. 'Medical Developments and Patient Unrest in the Leprosy Asylum, 1860–1940.' *Social Scientist* 24, no. 4/6, 65.
20. Moran, *Colonizing Leprosy*, 74–103; Stanley, Laurie C.C. 1995. '"So Many Crosses to Bear:" The Religious Hospitallers of St Joseph and the Tracadie Leper Hospital, 1868–1910.' In *Changing Roles of Women within the Christian Church in Canada*, ed. Elizabeth Gillan Muir and Marilyn Fardig Whiteley. Toronto: University of Toronto Press, 19–37; Ngoc Yen, L.H. 2018. 'The Nuns of Lepers: Compassion, Discipline and Surrogate Parenthood in a Former Leper Colony of Vietnam.' *The Asia Pacific Journal of Anthropology* 19 (4), 350–366; Vongsathorn, Kathleen. 2012. '"First and Foremost the Evangelist"? Mission and Government Priorities for the Treatment of Leprosy in Uganda, 1927–48.' *Journal of East African Studies* 6 (3), 544–560.
21. Brown, Raphael 1951. *World Survey of Catholic Leprosy Work*. Techny, Illinois: The Mission Press, SVD, 26.
22. Mann Wall, Barbra. 2015. *Into Africa: A Transnational History of Catholic Medical Missions and Social Change*. New Brunswick, New Jersey: Rutgers University Press, 8.
23. Gussow, *Leprosy, Racism and Public Health*, 208–211; Vaughan, *Curing Their Ills*; Sykes, Ingrid J. 2017. 'Humanitarian Quarantine in Practice: Medicine, Religion and Leprosy in New Caledonia.' *Anthropology and Medicine* 24 (3), 301–318; Bernabeu-Mestre and Ballester-Artigues, 'Disease as a Metaphorical Resource,' 409–421.
24. Mann Wall, *Into Africa*, 2.
25. Carey, 'Subordination, Invisibility and Chosen Work,' 252.

26. Nelson, Sioban. 2001. *Say Little, Do Much: Nursing, Nuns and Hospitals in the Nineteenth Century*. Philadelphia Pa:University of Pennsylvania Press, 13.
27. Gardiner, Ann. 2008. *The Flame In the North: The Daughters of Our Lady of the Sacred Heart 1908–2008*. Darwin: the author; Venard, Mary. 1974. *The History of the Australian Province of the Daughters of Our Lady of the Sacred Heart*. Kensington: *Daughters of Our Lady of the Sacred Heart*; Allen, Doris M. 1995. *Frank Flynn MSC: A Remarkable Territorian*, Kensington: Chevalier Press; Thomson, Ann. 1988. *NT Dreaming: The Story of the Catholic Church in the Northern Territory*. Darwin: Catholic Education Office; Durack, Mary. 1969. *The Rock and the Sand*. London: Constable & Co. Ltd.; Zucker, Margaret. 2005. *From Patrons to Partners And the Separated Children of the Kimberly: A History of the Catholic Church in the Kimberley* WA, second edition. Fremantle: University of Notre Dame Press; Scally, John. 1995. *To Speed on Angels' Wings: the Story of the Sisters of St John of God*. Dublin: The Columba Press; MacGinley, M.R. 2010. *An Eloquent Witness: The Sisters of Our Lady Help of Christians*. Strathfield: St Pauls Publications.
28. Zucker, *From Patrons to Partners*, 78–83; Thomson, *NT Dreaming*, 20.
29. Watego, *Another Day in the Colony*, 62.
30. Scollard, D.M., L.B. Adams, T.P. Gillis, J.L. Krahenbuhl, R.W. Truman, and D.L. Williams. 2006. 'The Continuing Challenges of Leprosy.' *Clinical Microbiology Review* 19 (2), 361.
31. Thompson, Paul. 2010. 'The Voice of the Past: Oral History.' In *The Oral History Reader*, second edition, ed. Robert Perks and Alistair Thomson, USA and Canada: Routledge, 28.
32. Garibaldi Rogers, Carole. 1998. 'Overlooked Narratives: What Women Religious Can Contribute to Feminist Oral History.' *Frontiers* 19 (3), 164–5, 168.
33. Portelli, Alessandro. 'What Makes Oral History Different.' In *The Oral History Reader*, ed. Perks and Thomson, 38.
34. Domachowske, Joseph and Manika, Suryadevara. 2020. 'Leprosy.' In: *Clinical Infectious Diseases Study Guide*. Springer, Cham. https://doi-org.wwwproxy1.library.unsw.edu.au/10.1007/978-3-030-50873-9_53. Accessed 20 Jan 2022; Northern Territory Medical Service. 1968. *Leprosy in Northern Territory Aborigines*. Darwin: Government Printer for Northern Territory Medical Service, 9–18.
35. Scollard et al. 'The Continuing Challenges of Leprosy,' 338–339, 347.
36. Anderson, *Colonial Pathologies*, 708, 715; Moran, *Colonizing Leprosy*, 49–51; Deacon, Harriet. 1996. 'Racial Segregation and Medical Discourse in Nineteenth-Century Cape Town.' *Journal of South African Studies* 22(2), 287–308.

37. Jebb, Mary Anne. 1984. 'The Lock Hospitals Experiment: Europeans, Aborigines and Venereal Disease.' In *European-Aboriginal Relations in Western Australian History*, ed. Bob Reece and Tom Stannage. Studies in Western Australian History, Nedlands: Department of History, University of Western Australia, 68–87; Parsons, Meg. 2008. 'Fantome Island Lock Hospital and Aboriginal Venereal Disease Sufferers, 1928–45.' *Health and History* 10 (1), 41–62.
38. Broome, Richard. 2010. *Aboriginal Australians: A History Since 1788*, fourth edition. Sydney: Allen and Unwin, 118–121; McGregor, Russell. 1998. *Imagined Destinies: Aboriginal Australians and the Doomed Race Theory 1880–1939.* Carlton: Melbourne University Press; Evans, Raymond. 1999. *Fighting Words: Writing about Race*. St Lucia: University of Queensland Press, 123–146.
39. Bashford, *Imperial Hygiene*, 98.
40. O'Brien, *Philanthropy and Settler Colonialism*, 110.

CHAPTER 2

Foundations

In the second half of the nineteenth century, long after leprosy had declined in most of Europe, the disease again found prominence for the Christian West with its spread to the colonised world. With the theory that leprosy was communicable gaining acceptance, isolation of sufferers remotely or on islands intensified. Leprosy, particularly in colonised countries, became linked with the non-European races, and exclusion aimed to contain those deemed unfit for the envisaged twentieth-century nation-state. Concomitantly, Christian missionary outreach from Europe brought leprosy sufferers into the stewardship of the religious, continuing the longstanding tradition of Christ's mandate for the care of the sick and abandoned, and the medieval Christians' reconceptualisation of the figure of the 'leper,' Molokai's Father Damien inspired modern missionaries with his religious and cultural evangelisation of the 'native leper.' Catholic Sisters partook in the global missionary enterprise. As nurses, were integral to leprosy institutions. In Australia, Christian Churches had no formal involvement in leprosy care before the late interwar period, their attention diverted to parishes and schools, and Sisters' teaching work was prioritised. Leprosy was treated as a disease of foreigners and its elimination from Australian shores took priority, through island detention or by deportation.

C. Robson, *Missionary Women, Leprosy and Indigenous Australians, 1936–1986*, https://doi.org/10.1007/978-3-031-05796-0_2

Christian Caregiving of Leprosy-Affected People in History

The care by Christian religious of leprosy sufferers in the modern age derives from a long tradition initiated in the teachings of the New Testament and developed over many centuries of Western European civilisation. In the Old Testament, 'leprosy' is depicted as a divine punishment for committing sin. 'Lepers' are considered 'unclean' and are exiled from society under the authority of the priest. If, after a period, the disease is healed, the 'leper' may be reincorporated into the community following repentance with the sacrifice of burnt offerings to God. The New Testament introduced the concept of Christian care-giving, exemplified in Christ's solicitude towards the outcast 'lepers' he encounters and promoted to his followers in his instruction to 'cleanse the lepers.' The idea that 'lepers' should be drawn into the society of Christians is extended in the parable of Lazarus whose suffering and social marginalisation led to sanctification and was rewarded with eternal salvation.

Assessing the treatment of leprosy sufferers in medieval Western Europe and Britain, some historians have agreed with Sheldon Watts, that Christians at this time saw the 'leper' as "a sin-curst being, who, following the precepts of Leviticus, must be cast out of the community of the faithful."[1] Parallels have been drawn between the ancient Mosaic ritual of social exclusion and the subjection of medieval leprosy sufferers to separation rites in which they are pronounced 'dead' and cruelly banished from society.[2] Later studies have shown that this view fails to account for the impact of the New Testament on what was a deeply devout Christian society. Medievalist Carole Rawcliffe has argued that "a belief that confirmed lepers should live 'outside the camp' did not condemn them to banishment or neglect."[3] She demonstrates that conditions of the medieval monastic leprosaria reflected the perception by Christians that the 'leper' occupied a special status, as one close to God. Rawcliffe challenges perceptions that religious custody was necessarily inconsistent with therapeutic care. Although leprosy was incurable in the Middle Ages, medical treatments were attempted and other supportive measures implemented for palliative or cosmetic purposes, or for immediate relief.[4]

The Christian conceptualisation of the 'leper' as the simultaneous embodiment of abjectness and sanctity was demonstrated most clearly in hagiographies of the medieval saint, Francis of Assisi, published from the late nineteenth to early twentieth century. His original repulsion on encountering a 'leper' quickly changes to humility and deference as he recognises Christ manifest in the man before him. Francis promptly exchanges his hedonistic ways and material riches for the life of an impoverished mendicant and spends much of his time in the leper-houses, bathing the sores of the inmates, and becoming, himself, spiritually enriched. [5] The biographies of Francis illustrate further portrayals of leprosy and other illnesses, not as a punishment for sin as histories have argued was the Christian perception, but as a divine bestowal. To the 'leper' who was disillusioned with a God who "has made my body a mass of stinking and corruption," Francis said, "My brother, be patient, for God gives us diseases in this world for the salvation of souls, and when we endure them patiently, they are a fountain of great merit to us."[6]

These familiar strands of Christian charity, with the 'leper' as a symbol for the suffering and outcast, formed the basis of the apostolate for Francis' new order of male religious, the Friars Minor. Traditional monks in this period remained in their cloisters, dedicated to prayer and contemplation, working towards their own sanctification—the first duty of every professed religious. The Franciscans broke with this convention in practising a new form of ascetism that blended monastic piety with Christian philanthropy without compromising self-sanctification.[7] The Friars Minor rapidly expanded to become an international society in Francis' own time. Their guiding philosophy and way of life was, in one way or another, the inspiration for every Christian religious with an active apostolate.

In this context, premodern religious Sisters took up the dispensing of services to the sick and poor as an intrinsic part of their vocation, but it was a right they had to continually defend until the nineteenth century. The Roman Church frowned upon the active apostolate for women, insisting that Sisters who professed the solemn and perpetual vows of chastity, poverty, and obedience remain confined to their cloisters. Women attempted to circumvent these restrictions, by working clandestinely or forming their own simple-vowed ('Third Order') communities, such as the Sisters of the Holy Ghost who founded the Hotel Dieu in Paris. Included in the nursing work of this group and others in the Middle Ages was the care of leprosy sufferers, indicating a long genealogy of the association of women religious with this work.[8]

A vigorous expansion in Christian evangelical activity in the middle of the nineteenth century brought missionaries of all denominations from

Europe into the overseas colonial mission fields. Catholic European religious congregations whose numbers swelled in the nineteenth century followed their Protestant counterparts into this venture, encouraged by the Vatican. They included active orders of vowed women religious who were granted papal approbation for the first time in 1816.[9] In what sociologist Zachary Gussow has called 'the separatist tradition,' the care and support of leprosy sufferers fell almost exclusively to missionaries.[10] Their involvement ranged from fund-raising ventures, such as that of the Mission to Lepers, to supervisory and pastoral roles, to complete institutional nursing and administration by communities of women religious. The care of leprosy sufferers by religious was not new.[11] What distinguished the movement after the middle of the nineteenth century was its pervasiveness across the globe, its formal organisation by bodies such as the Mission to Lepers, and the accompanying focus on the evangelisation of non-Christian races. This practice reflected the intersection of missionary motivations with the imperatives of modern health bureaucracies which, in many cases, through the confinement of leprosy sufferers in leprosaria without adequate arrangements for their support, had created abandoned populations in need of care. While missionaries may have identified them with biblical and medieval 'lepers,' as Gussow has contended, we cannot make assumptions about their perceptions or the implications for their welfare. Certainly, under drastic state policies of segregation, modern leprosy sufferers were outcast, very much in the way their earlier antecedents were imagined; this in itself invited Christian charity.

Inspiration for the care of modern leprosy sufferers can also be found in the narratives of esteemed religious figures. The story of Francis of Assisi was retold in several new publications in the late nineteenth and early twentieth centuries. They drew widespread interest, but, taken literally, they were especially relevant for those working with leprosy sufferers.[12] The modern Christian leprosy apostolate, set against the imperial missionary enterprise, was most comprehensively embodied in Father (later, Saint) Damien of the Kalaupapa 'leper colony' on the Hawaiian island of Molokai who was feted in the international press of his own time, and apotheosised in published biographies. He belonged to one of the French religious congregations established in the early nineteenth century which broadened its home apostolate to include evangelisation in the islands of the Pacific. To contemporary and later cohorts of Christian missionaries of this same tradition, his life story contextualised the examples of Francis of Assisi, and of Jesus Christ.[13]

Whereas Francis effected the renewal of Christian faith in his 'lepers,' Damien worked to convert the 'lepers' to Christianity and to bring about their cultural evangelisation. On arrival at Kalaupapa as parish priest in 1873, Damien reportedly found the residents in a state of abject misery, their huts insufficient shelter, and sores festering. He expressed disgust at the unregulated sex, excessive drinking, and poor church attendances. According to his biographies, Damien then took practical tasks to hand, building houses, cleaning wounds, and organising a fresh water supply. He also supposedly effected their spiritual transformation and created order from chaos, Christians from heathens, and respectability from moral degeneracy.[14]

Self-sacrifice was a compelling element of Damien's mission. Echoing St Francis' horror at his initial sight of the 'lepers,' Damien recalled in 1885 how the odours of the patients' ulcers had so assailed him at first that he took to smoking a pipe.[15] His ultimate sacrifice was contracting leprosy himself, an event that sealed his public image as a great martyr and, in confirming the inherent risk of contagion, stamped the leprosy apostolate as a work of deep unselfish devotion.[16] The parallels between Damien's affliction and the idea of Christ-as-leper embedded in Franciscan discourse deepened the significance of his work in the Christian world.

As well as glorifying the imperial leprosy apostolate, Damien's work also had the effect, as Pennie Moblo has pointed out, of constructing a particular stereotype of the Hawaiian leprosy sufferer.[17] Generated from the highly publicised Molokai leprosarium, this image came to define the 'native leper' globally. Without Damien's transformative work, the 'native lepers' seemed trapped in a spiral of physical and spiritual decline, apparent victims of their own ignorance, immorality, and lawlessness.[18] The state authorities had abandoned them and only through Damien's intervention could conditions be improved at the leper colony. The residents were thus portrayed as irresponsible and childlike, but also responsive and grateful for such Christian paternalism.[19] On such an image hinged the assumption that became crucial to the promotion of the Christian leprosy apostolate: the missionary was needed by the 'native leper.'

Coinciding with Damien's period at Kalaupapa, growing numbers of Catholic women religious acquired nursing positions in state leprosaria across the colonised world. This was a practice that became a dominant model of nursing care and general administration for late nineteenth to mid-twentieth century institutions worldwide. Early examples in the imperial West were Cocorite in Trinidad and Tracadie in New Brunswick, both of which acquired religious nursing staff in 1868. From the late 1880s until the early twentieth century, the leprosaria at Kalaupapa, Carville, Culion,and Makogai followed suit. Leprosy nursing in the years prior to antibiotic therapy aimed to ameliorate the effects of the disease, particularly in treating skin lesions with bandaging, cleansing, and applying salves and to provide general care such as feeding and bathing incapacitated individuals. After the turn of the twentieth century, Sisters administered the drug, chaulmoogra oil, the standard treatment internationally for leprosy at the time. Some Sisters tried out various experimental agents and assisted in medical research projects investigating disease transmission.[20]

By the late nineteenth century, the precedent set by Catholic religious Sisters in leprosarium nursing work was known internationally and they were seen as a valuable resource by governments seeking efficient and inexpensive ways of providing nursing care for those segregated in leprosaria. In Fiji, for example, the governor decided to staff Makogai with missionary Sisters in 1911 after hearing of the leprosy work begun four decades previously by the Dominican Sisters at Trinidad.[21] The few studies examining religious Sisters' work in the leprosaria attest to their assuming far greater responsibility over the lives of the inmates than supplying nursing services. The imposition of discipline, the inculcation of moral and religious values, instruction in handicrafts, organising work schedules, and general administration were some of the tasks they undertook, echoing the model set by Father Damien.[22] This overall reform was a kind of evangelisation, with more chance of success in the leprosarium, where patients were in many cases detained, and away from other, competing influences.

Christian Missions in Australia

Evangelical missionary societies, such as the London Missionary Society, established the first Christian mission stations in Australia, beginning in New South Wales in the 1820s. Following the tracks of European settlement, further stations were opened north and south along the east coast. But, within twenty years, all had closed after problems with attracting or maintaining contact with Indigenous people, or due to internal friction.[23]

In the second half of the nineteenth century, the Moravians and the Church of England established mission stations in South Australia and Victoria. Set up in the wake of rapid incursions by white settlers, they were encouraged and supported by governments seeking to minimise frontier violence.[24] For the Indigenous people who gathered at the Hagernauers' station, Ramahyuck, in Victoria's Gippsland, dispossession of their land had left them, according to Bain Attwood, "eking out a meagre existence" and therefore dependent on the mission for their physical survival.[25] At Poonindie in South Australia, Indigenous people also came voluntarily, some having been deprived of food supplies.[26] The mission founders aimed to convert them to Christianity and to acculturate them to Western culture and social values. They chose sites that were isolated from European settlers and Indigenous traditional lands to insulate their charges against influences that might undermine their own training programmes. Indigenous people were expected to conform to the nineteenth-century Victorian ideal of respectable domesticity, hard work and devout Christianity. The glaring exception was that their children were to be raised separately in boarding houses.

Poonindie and Ramahyuck, despite their harsh and alien conditions, became the centres of new Indigenous communities drawn together in agricultural self-sufficiency, Christian rituals, and the schooling of their children.[27] After the 1880s, government support for these missions was reduced, either through the protection acts, or by the sale of mission lands to private owners. Many Indigenous people in the south faced either tighter control on government reserves or had to seek work in a labour market squeezed by the economic recession and the endemic racial discrimination of the 1890s.[28]

Almost all nineteenth-century Catholic missionary ventures were quickly aborted, marked by severe disappointment, early abandonment of mission stations, and, sometimes, tragedy. All were led by priests from Europe with scarce support from their Church. Being in remote inhospitable regions, they presented enormous emotional and physical challenges. Examples were the Italian Passionists on Stradbroke Island, Queensland, begun in 1843; the French Jesuits in the Northern Territory, first at Daly River, then at Rapid Creek, during the last decades of the nineteenth century; and, in the same period, a fledgling mission in Derby, Western Australia also failed.[29] The notable exception was New Norcia in south-west Western Australia, founded in 1846 by Spanish Benedictine monk, Rosendo Salvado, which lasted for over 120 years.

The Australian Catholic Church in the nineteenth and early twentieth centuries was mostly interested in consolidating Catholicism for the settler population in a country dominated by British Protestantism. The bishops, who, after the 1860s, were for the most part, Irishmen, directed episcopal funds and the energies of the religious to the growing parishes of white Catholics, also predominantly Irish-born or of Irish extraction. Irish priests continued to dominate the senior echelons of the Australian clergy well into the middle of the twentieth century, reinforcing the same values and priorities. When a prestigious seminary was established in Manly in 1885 for Australian-born aspirants, it was with the Catholic parish in mind, not the mission fields.[30] Therefore, neither opportunities nor encouragement were offered for men to pursue an Australian missionary vocation.

European Catholic missionary orders of male religious in Australia in this period prioritised overseas missions. In 1885, the Missionaries of the Sacred Heart (MSC) arrived from France to set up a base for their Pacific missions and, two years later, founded a missionary college in Kensington, Sydney to prepare men to "go forth to work in distant lands."[31] The Pacific Islands, Asia and Africa were the "real foreign missions," known for their large vibrant communities and embrace of the Christian message, making a missionary's industry and sacrifice worthwhile.[32] For these missionaries, Indigenous Australians were on the verge of extinction or incapable of responding to Catholic missionaries' evangelising efforts.[33]

In 1901 the Pallottines, a German Catholic men's order, established an Indigenous mission at Beagle Bay in the Kimberley region of Western Australia. Ten years later, Francis Xavier Gsell MSC began a mission with the Tiwi people on Bathurst Island, off the Northern Territory coast.[34] These missions reflected increased interest by Christian missionaries of all denominations in northern coastal Indigenous people in the first half of the twentieth century. An interdenominational agreement was reached in 1912, allocating to each group a particular geographical sphere of influence within the area north of 20° south latitude. The distribution was based on the locations of existing missions to avoid the overlap of competing operations. In the following decades, the different missionary organisations added new mission stations to their original holdings. To some extent, patterns of Indigenous Christian belief in the twenty-first century reflect the original divisions.[35] The Catholic Church in the far north-east coast of the Northern Territory expanded from the original Bathurst Island station to include Melville Island, Port Keats, and

Daly River; to the Beagle Bay mission in the Kimberley, La Grange and Lombadina were added. The Church of England which owned Roper River Mission, was granted control of eastern Arnhem Land where it added Groote Eylandt and Oenpelli Missions, while in Queensland, south of the Cape York Peninsula, Edward and Lockhart Rivers missions were added to the older stations at Yarrabah and Mitchell River. Similar patterns were followed by the other denominations, notwithstanding the gradual incursions of organisations such as the United Aborigines Mission.

The protection policy discussed in Chapter 1, took place for many Indigenous people, on these northern missions. The Doomed Race Theory persisted in the early half of the twentieth century, but, increasingly, missionaries, as well as some anthropologists and government officials subscribed to the view that the Indigenous races could survive if removed from the influence of nefarious Europeans to the Christianising and 'civilising' projects of the missions.[36] Some missions acted as havens for Indigenous people who, due to European incursions on their lands, had lost food and water sources and been subjected to diseases and settler violence. On the colonial frontiers, missionaries were among the few to provide health care to Indigenous people by providing basic medical relief, nutrition, and physical safety.[37] Gsell, who had no medical qualifications dispensed remedies, performed dental procedures, and extracted spears from wounds, as did Bishop Salvado at New Norcia. Bishop Raible of Beagle Bay employed medically qualified personnel from Europe as resident mission physicians. Implicit in this medical care was an assumption that their medicine was superior, just as they firmly believed their religion and culture to be. How effective the unqualified medical care was, or how it influenced the attitude of the Indigenous people they attended is unknown, but it is probable that some success contributed to the paternal image of these European mission leaders who first drew the curious and hungry to their mission doors.[38]

Yet, the physical health of Indigenous people on missions could not always be assured. Food and health care were sometimes abysmally inadequate, either through negligence or the mission's own deprivations. Infectious diseases quickly took hold when people, once living in smaller more mobile groups, were concentrated together.[39] However, some historians suggest that 'protection' as a strategy for survival on missions and reserves ultimately succeeded as Indigenous populations increased over the first half of the twentieth century.[40]

The Emergence of Catholic Mission Sisters in Australia

In the first years following European settlement, the Church of England was the only denomination to receive recognition and support, and the Catholic Church struggled to stake its claim in the colonies. Of particular concern to Bishop John Bede Polding in New South Wales was the condition of the sick and poor in the colony, especially among Irish migrants. One strategy was to invite religious Sisters from Ireland where a revitalisation of the Catholic orders was in progress. Centuries of religious oppression, beginning with Henry VIII's dissolution of the monastic houses through to the imposition of a series of penal codes in the eighteenth century, had left the Irish Catholic apostolate relatively quiescent until the Catholic Emancipation of 1829. Thereafter many new congregations were formed, reflecting the burgeoning of single Irish women ready to commit themselves to the expression of their faith through charitable works and perpetual devotion to God.[41]

The first female religious to arrive were teachers and nurses of the Irish Sisters of Charity, a congregation formed as an offshoot of the French Soeurs de Charité. These women, who established St. Vincent's Hospital in Sydney in 1857, were largely responsible for cementing the reputation of religious nursing Sisters in Australia as skilled, capable, and pioneering practitioners. In a period when few nurses were professionally trained, many Sisters of Charity received nurse training at the highly respected St. Vincent's Hospital in Paris, where apart from professional skills, they adopted habits such as discipline and neatness, that later became synonymous with general nursing practices. The Australian Sisters were known for treating anyone who required their care, regardless of religious affiliations, and seem not to have engaged in overt proselytisation—characteristics that doubtless stood them in good stead among Australian society generally.[42] Catholic Sisters of the Irish congregations, the Sisters of Mercy and the Sisters of St John of God, founded a further nine hospitals in the colonies before the century closed.[43]

By far more numerous than the nurses were the Irish and European religious teaching Sisters recruited in the drive by the Australian Church, first, to provide Catholic high school education and then, through the 1870s and 1880s, to staff primary schools following the withdrawal of state aid to denominational schools. The Sisters were valued for their dedicated, unpaid work, and for a teaching ethos and curriculum steeped in Western European tradition, arising from the education and training of Irish Catholic women in France. The identity of the Irish Sisters also reassured the families of their pupils as they shared a past of an Ireland besieged by famine, Protestant intolerance, and British colonialism. Catholic schools, by educating and bolstering the community, were a safeguard against the possibility of such oppression in the context of the British colonies in Australia.[44]

The placement of religious Sisters in Catholic education services was an important factor in the growth of religious sectarianism. Despite the integration of many Catholics into mainstream Australian society, there remained a sense that some clustered together defensively under the umbrella of Irish Catholic nationalism. The perception—real or suspected—of Catholic clannishness predicated on an agenda disparate to the common Australian cause underlay a persistent divisiveness in Australian society, resurfacing particularly in times of national crises. Catholics who opposed the proposed conscription in World War 1, the interning of German Catholic priests, and the proposal of taxing bachelors who did not enlist—the last two seen as singling out male religious—were seen as disloyal and sectarian.[45]

Under official church rules, women were prohibited from initiating their own missions, a prerogative of a senior priest or bishop, whose religious congregation was authorised for mission work in a particular geographic region by the Vatican's Propaganda del Fide. Catholic Sisters usually entered the Australian Indigenous mission fields by invitation of the local bishop in his role as apostolic head, in recognition that women were essential for a mission's success. One reason was their ability to attract otherwise wary Indigenous women and young children to mission stations, an important factor since children past puberty were deemed less responsive to evangelisation.[46]

Catholic Sisters transformed the Indigenous missions into domestic spaces, suitable for accommodating removed children. As females, even under religious vows, they were assumed to be natural housekeepers and mothers, and many were trained and/or experienced nurses and teachers.[47] They were vital to the "planting of a living 'slice' of Europeanization," through the gendered segregation of education and training. [48] Brothers and priests taught the boys carpentry, stock work, and mechanics while Sisters taught the girls dressmaking and cooking in preparation for survival in the encroaching white Western society. They encouraged marriages among mission residents with the aim of creating devout and hardworking Catholic families. Sisters set and defended this moral order through their supervision and training of young Indigenous females. In the Kimberley, the Sisters deplored the trade of sex with girls for tobacco or money by local pearlers, and it became justification for their removal to the Catholic orphanage.[49]

Leprosy in Australia 1850s to 1920s

By the sixteenth century, the leprosy epidemics of medieval England and Western Europe had largely subsided, but the disease continued to affect populations of outlying countries such as Ireland until the mid-eighteenth century and Finland, Norway, and Spain, until the late nineteenth century.[50] Its appearance in the Americas and the Caribbean islands from the sixteenth century have been attributed to European colonisation and the slave trade from West Africa where leprosy had long been endemic. The disease has a proven long history in India and China also. When contemporaries became aware of leprosy during the nineteenth century in Oceania, including in Hawaii, Fiji, New Zealand, and Australia, they assumed it was newly introduced and had been spread by Chinese indentured labourers—a theory that has been reiterated in later epidemiological studies and histories. Twenty-first century DNA researchers, however, have concluded that the disease had been present in Pacific islands for much longer, and probably arrived in waves of human migration thousands of years earlier, although they do not rule out re-introductions of leprosy through the recent colonisation of the Pacific by Europeans.[51] Australia has not had a parallel study, therefore the data available on its early history of leprosy relies on empirical observation by contemporaries, sources that can only provide an incomplete picture.

John Ashburton Thompson was one epidemiologist who was aware of the inadequacies of the available data when, in 1894, he investigated leprosy in Australia. He thus came to no definite conclusions. The absence of reported leprosy cases among Indigenous people prior to the 1880s did not convince him that the 'autochthons,' as he called pre-contact Indigenous, had been free of the disease. Nor was he persuaded of the argument common in his day that white Australians with leprosy in the south must have contracted it from afflicted Chinese people. The reports of white cases soon after the arrival of the latter was no proof, and could have been coincidental, he argued. Thompson's monograph was written just two years after the first notifications of Indigenous people with leprosy to

Australian health authorities. Only a trickle of cases had emerged—in the south-east and far north of Queensland (Maryborough and Townsville respectively) and around the Alligator River in the northern reaches of the Northern Territory. Again, because he could not find absolute proof, Thompson believed it unlikely that leprosy was contagious. If it was, he posited, surely more Indigenous people would have contracted it after years of contact with outsiders, including the Macassans on the north coast for hundreds of years previously. Over the ensuing years, they did. Increases not only occurred in the areas mentioned, but new cases appeared in places such as Cairns and Mackay in Queensland, and Arnhem Land in the Northern Territory. Around 1907, the first Indigenous cases came to light in Western Australia, at pastoral stations in the Roebourne area.[52]

Thompson's monograph traced the earliest recorded cases in Australia to the middle of the nineteenth century among Chinese goldminers in Victoria. This outbreak had not led to any official action. In the 1880s, an increase in cases, almost all of whom were Chinese, was reported in New South Wales, Queensland, and the Northern Territory.[53] Respective colonial governments acted to remove the few suspected leprosy sufferers from proximity to the Australian public, to island lazarets in the northern colonies, or, in New South Wales, beachside huts below the Coast Hospital at Little Bay. Isolation was intended to be temporary, and most were eventually deported to their home countries of China or Hong Kong.[54] Conditions at Mud Island in the Northern Territory and Dayman Island off the coast of far north Queensland, both of which received Chinese leprosy suspects from 1889, reveal a picture of utter despair. Without essentials for survival, many perished—if not through illness or starvation, then by their own hand.[55] Their fate made the attitudes of governments painfully clear: leprosy was a foreign disease—specifically a Chinese disease—and its elimination from Australian shores was imperative, irrespective of the cost to its victims.

The removals of Chinese people in the late nineteenth century occurred against a rising tide of anti-Chinese sentiment. Some politicians and sections of the press blamed the Chinese for spreading smallpox in New South Wales during the 1881 epidemic, leading to their victimisation and the passage of immigration restriction legislation.[56] By the late 1880s, as leprosy became of concern overseas and in the Australian colonies, the Chinese were again blamed for importing yet another disease. In New

South Wales, a newspaper advised prohibiting Chinese ownership of property for fear that "Leprosy might be harboured for months in the Chinese warrens" and another, in Queensland, claimed that the Chinese were "saturated with leprosy germs."[57] These publications represented workers' rights, the broader context being the economically unstable 1890s during which the Chinese were accused of undercutting white men's wages and taking their jobs. The vitriolic and sometimes violent campaigns against the Chinese were based on the claim to a British settler identity and the privileging of the rights of the white working male.[58] Both would become inscribed in foundational policies of the newly federated nation after 1901, most explicitly the White Australia policy and the 'living wage.'

Pacific Islanders, first reported with leprosy in the 1890s, excited similar anxieties, particularly in Queensland. Having arrived years before as indentured labourers to work the sugar cane-fields of northern New South Wales and southern Queensland, this group had become unpopular with the white working class, due to competition for work and to entrenched racism.[59] As it became more evident to Australian health authorities that leprosy was a communicable disease, Pacific Islanders and the Chinese loomed large as the transmitters of the disease in the eyes of many white Australians including doctors and health boards. Leprosy, like smallpox and competitive labour, represented a threat by non-white migrants to a healthy, prosperous white citizenry and provided another reason for expelling these races, whether through lazaret isolation, deportation, or immigration restriction.[60]

Measures by Australian governments to deal with leprosy reflected not only local concerns and conditions, but circulating ideas and policies overseas, especially in the British Empire. Despite the presence of the disease among the peoples of the world's northernmost countries, Iceland and Norway, many doctors and colonial government administrators of the mid to late nineteenth century defined leprosy as a disease of the tropics, contracted by the dark-skinned inhabitants, through heredity or environmental factors. It seemed that leprosy posed no real threat to citizens of the Western metropolis, and indeed, the view of some administrators directly confronting the disease in colonies such as the Cape and British Guiana was that leprosy was not contagious. However, in 1865, Hawaiian authorities, convinced that Chinese migrants had infected the indigenous people with leprosy introduced compulsory segregation for sufferers on the island of Molokai. The identification of a causative bacillus by Norwegian microbiologist, Gerhard-Henrik Armauer Hansen in 1873 added weight to the theory of contagion. The Royal College of Physicians, however, remained committed to their anti-contagionist stance, even in the mid-1880s when Father Damien, the Belgian missionary priest of Molokai, fell ill with leprosy.[61] The contagion theory thereafter grew momentum, culminating in what Zachary Gussow has called "the peak years of panic in Great Britain" (the late 1880s to the mid-1890s).[62] Laws enacting compulsory segregation swept through much of the imperial world, for example, in British Columbia, the Philippines, Fiji, and Cape Colony, with the result that thousands of leprosy sufferers were detained in 'leper colonies' until well into the next century.[63]

Records of white people with leprosy in Australia date back to the 1860s and 1870s in New South Wales and Queensland. These cases were seen by doctors, and some were admitted to hospitals for short periods then released. All were assumed to have contracted the disease overseas.[64] A decade later, health authorities began receiving notifications of white leprosy sufferers who had never travelled outside Australia, suggesting local transmissions. In response, New South Wales passed the *Leprosy Act* (1890) which made the notification of leprosy sufferers compulsory and empowered officials to enforce their isolation. The Governor was granted the authority to set aside any site as a lazaret. Queensland followed suit in 1892.[65] Other colonies amended or used existing public health laws as the need arose. Non-white people had been isolated without such laws for some years, a practice that was clearly thought unacceptable for white leprosy sufferers. The outcomes for the latter were, however, variable. In New South Wales, most people with leprosy, regardless of race, were admitted to the aforementioned Little Bay lazaret near Sydney. Queensland had a specific lazaret for white people on Stradbroke Island in Moreton Bay until 1907, when it opened a leprosarium on Peel Island for all races. Here, the patients were segregated according to race and gender, the white patients living in measurably more comfortable conditions and with better food than the 'coloured' patients. But white Queensland leprosy sufferers detained on the island lazarets were not spared the misery endured by their non-white counterparts. And if race did not save a person from this fate, class sometimes did. Middle- to upper-class white people diagnosed with leprosy were more likely to arouse the sympathy of doctors or health boards, and many either escaped official notification or were permitted to isolate at home.[66]

For many Indigenous people, as well as some Chinese and Pacific Islanders, removal and confinement from the late nineteenth century were brutal experiences. Often, they were restrained at various places until transport to a lazaret could be arranged. The police, who usually had the job of collecting prospective patients from their homes, sometimes held them in tents in police paddocks, as Hugo Rée has discussed with regard to Queensland. At times, individual policemen, apparently struck by the hardship endured by their charges, performed small acts of kindness, such as supplying them with tobacco or other "luxuries."[67] At Broome in Western Australia, Indigenous leprosy-affected people were held at the local police paddock in the early part of the twentieth century.[68] When Indigenous detainees proved difficult to confine, police or doctors resorted to using chains. A Queensland man, Jerry, was confirmed as having leprosy in March 1914, and held at Leper Point near Cairns, pending removal to Peel Island leprosarium. A government report stated that since "Jerry is a wild black…we have to keep him chained up," and there he remained until he died, seven months later.[69] Leg irons were still being used to secure patients in 1929, and chains continued to be used on Indigenous patients in Western Australia up to the late 1940s.[70]

The early removals of Indigenous people were nearly all to islands: Mud Island (Northern Territory); Friday Island from the 1890s followed by Dayman Island (Queensland); and Bezout Island from 1910, followed by Cossack on the mainland (Western Australia). On arrival at the lazarets, the people faced conditions that gave away only too clearly the purpose of their removal. The remoteness that segregated the healthy from the diseased also separated the inmates from almost every form of available support and care. All the islands were deficient in water, firewood, and food supplies, so the inmates had to rely on deliveries from the mainland. Being situated in areas subjected to recurrent tropical cyclones and other extreme weather, visits to the islands often had to be delayed or cancelled. Medical attention by doctors was occasionally provided but severely hindered by access difficulties as well as personnel shortages due to the aversion of working in remote Australia. Before the mid-1920s, there were no resident caretakers, and inmates often had to build their own accommodation.[71] Unsurprisingly, many of the early inhabitants died within a short time of their incarceration.[72]

By the early 1920s, the proportion of Chinese and Pacific Islanders in Australian lazarets had decreased due to death or deportation. Furthermore, fewer of these cases had come to light due to the immigration restriction legislation enacted under the Commonwealth government's White Australia policy. European notifications had increased as had

Indigenous ones, the latter almost all of whom were found in Queensland, the Northern Territory, and north-west Western Australia.[73] By this period, Queensland Indigenous cases were detained at the Peel Island leprosarium while Mud Island continued as the lazaret in the Northern Territory, despite increasing criticism of its poor conditions. In Western Australia, most, if not all, the Cossack patients had died and a new outbreak had occurred among Indigenous people in Derby and Broome. Because transport to Cossack was costly and difficult, the former home of the Derby doctor, known as the 'old Residency'—a dilapidated weatherboard house—was used as a lazaret.[74] But at this moment, leprosy, and the people it affected—or might affect—began to capture the interest of Australians outside these far-flung corners of the country. Leprosy would soon find its way into the business of federal and state government administrators, senior medical officers, and missionaries.

Notes

1. Watts, Sheldon. 1997. *Epidemics and History: Disease, Power, and Imperialism*. New Haven & London: Yale University Press, 52.
2. Ibid., 46; Brody, Saul Nathaniel. 1974. *The Disease of the Soul: Leprosy in Medieval Literature*. Ithaca and London: Cornell University Press, 104–106.
3. Rawcliffe, Carole. 2006. *Leprosy in Medieval England*. Woodbridge: Boydell Press, 256.
4. Ibid., 56–63, 241; Risse, Guenter B. 1999. *Mending Bodies, Saving Souls: A History of Hospitals*. New York: Oxford University Press, 188–189; Demaitre, Luke. 2007. *Leprosy in Premodern Medicine: A Malady of the Whole Body*. Baltimore: John Hopkins University Press, 260–277.
5. St Francis quoted in 'Francis and Minority: Spirituality,' *Franciscan Friars: Province of the Holy Spirit*, www.franciscans.org.au/spirituality/minority.html, accessed 22 Dec 2010.
6. Sabatier, Paul and Jon M. Sweeney. 2003. *The Road to Assisi: The Essential Biography of St. Francis*. Brewster: Paraclete Press, 67.
7. Mrs Oliphant. 1889. Francis of Assisi. London and New York: MacMillan and Co., 67–68; McBrien, Richard P. 1980. *Catholicism*, volume two. Victoria: Dove Communications, 623.
8. Carey, Hilary M. 1998. 'Subordination, Invisibility and Chosen Work: Missionary Nuns and Australian Aborigines c.1900–1949.' *Australian Feminist Studies* 13 (28), 253; McNamara, Jo Ann Kay. 1996. *Sisters in Arms: Catholic Nuns Through Two Millennia*. Massachusetts: Harvard University Press, 142–143, 317, 461–462; Rapley, Elizabeth. 1990. *The*

Devotes: Women and Church in Seventeenth-century France. Montreal: McGill-Queen's University Press, 5, 24–28.

9. McNamara, *Sisters in Arms*, 583; Hogan, Edmund M. 1992. *The Irish Missionary Movement: A Historical Survey 1830–1980*. Dublin: Gill and Macmillan, 55–56, 59.
10. Gussow, Zachary. 1989. *Leprosy Racism & Public Health: Social Policy in Chronic Disease Control*. Boulder: Westview Press, 21.
11. E.g. the Philippines, mid-sixteenth century; Rio de Janeiro, 1760s; and Norway, early nineteenth century: Jarcho, S. 1973. 'Medical Numismatic Notes, ix: Coins of the Leper Colony at Culion and of the Philippine Health Service.' *Bulletin of the New York Academy of Medicine* 49 (2), 156; International Leprosy Association, Global Project on the History of Leprosy, *Timeline*, http://www.Leprosyhistory.org/cgi-bin/timelocsubbrowse.pl. Accessed 14 February 2012.
12. Moblo, Penny. 1997. 'Blessed Damien of Moloka'i: the Critical Analysis of Contemporary Myth.' *Ethnohistory* 44 (4), 702–3.
13. Ibid., 702; Edmond, Rod. 2006. *Leprosy and Empire: A Medical and Cultural History*. New York: Cambridge University Press, 93, 151–152.
14. Dutton, Charles J. 1932. *The Samaritans of Molokai*. New York: Dodd, Mead & Co., 71–78; Moblo, 'Blessed Damien,' 703–706.
15. de Veuster, Joseph. 1886. Report to Board of Health cited in Dutton, *The Samaritans of Molokai,* 66.
16. Edmond, *Leprosy and Empire*, 91.
17. Moblo, 'Blessed Damien,' 71.
18. Nineteenth century American protestant missionaries viewed Hawaiians in similar terms See Herman, R.D.K. 2001. 'Out of Sight, Out of Mind, Out of Power: Leprosy, Race and Colonization in Hawaii.' *Journal of Historical Geography* 27 (3), 322.
19. Moblo, 'Blessed Damien,' 702, 715.
20. Moran, Michelle T. 2007. *Colonising Leprosy: Imperialism and the Politics of Public Health in the United States*. Chapel Hill: University of North Carolina Press, 81; Stanley, Laurie C.C. 1995. '"So Many Crosses to Bear": The Religious Hospitallers of St Joseph and the Tracadie Leper Hospital, 1868–1910.' In *Changing Roles of Women within the Christian Church in Canada*, ed. Elizabeth Gillan Muir and Marilyn Fardig Whiteley. Toronto: University of Toronto Press, 37; Mary Stella SMSM, Sr. 1978. *Makogai: Image of Hope*, New Zealand: Lepers Trust Board Inc., 49; de Verteuil, F.A. and Fernand L. de Verteuil. 1912. 'Bacillus Lepra in the Nasal Mucosa.' *Canadian Medical Association Journal* 2 (1), 13.
21. Sir Everard im Thurn quoted in Sister Stella, *Makogai*, 34–35.
22. Gould, Tony 2005. *Don't Fence Me In: From Curse to Cure. Leprosy in Modern Times*. London: Bloomsbury, 32–33; Moran, *Colonizing Leprosy*, 102; Sister Stella, *Makogai*, 56; Stanley, 'So Many Crosses,' 33.

23. O'Brien, Anne. 2015. *Philanthropy and Settler Colonialism*. Basingstoke: Palgrave Macmillan, 31–32.
24. Brock, Peggy. 1993. *Outback Ghettoes: A History of Aboriginal Institutionalisation and Survival*. Cambridge: Cambridge University Press, 24, 27; Harris, John. 1990. *One Blood: Two Hundred Years of Aboriginal Encounter with Christianity: A Story of Hope*. Sutherland: Albatross Books, 173, 176, 200, 341.
25. Attwood, Bain. 1989. *The Making of the Aborigines*. Sydney: Allen and Unwin, 2.
26. Brock, *Outback Ghettoes*, 37.
27. Raftery, Judith. 2006. *Not Part of the Public: Non-indigenous policies and practices and the health of indigenous South Australians 1836–1973*. Kent Town: Wakefield Press, 107–108; Attwood, *The Making of the Aborigines*, 41–42.
28. Brock, *Outback Ghettoes*, 55–59; Broome, Richard. 2010. *Aboriginal Australians: A History Since 1788*, fourth edition. Sydney: Allen and Unwin, 94, 98.
29. Ganter, Regina. 2018. *The Contest for Aboriginal Souls: European Missionary Agendas in Australia*. Australian Capital Territory: ANU Press, 12–20, 54–55.
30. Livingstone, K.T. 1977. *The Emergence of an Australian Catholic Priesthood 1835–1915*. Sydney: Catholic Theological Faculty, xiv-xv, 101; Turner, Naomi. 1992. *Catholics in Australia: A Social History*, volume one. North Blackburn: Collins Dove, 89.
31. Moran, Archbishop Patrick, quoted in *Annals of our Lady of the Sacred Heart*, January 1, 1898, 33.
32. Broome, *Aboriginal Australians*, 152, 164.
33. Girola, Stefano. 2007. Rhetoric and Action: The Policies and Attitudes of the Catholic Church with regard to Australia's Indigenous Peoples 1885–1967. Ph.D. Diss. University of Queensland, 38–43.
34. Ganter, *The Contest for Aboriginal Souls*, 60, 138.
35. Arthur, Bill and Frances Morphy. 2005. *Macquarie Atlas of Indigenous Australia: Culture and Society Through Space and Time*. NSW: The Macquarie Library Pty Ltd, 103–107; Harris, *One Blood*, 689, 725.
36. McGregor, Russell. 1998. *Imagined Destinies: Aboriginal Australians and the Doomed Race Theory 1880–1939*. Carlton South: Melbourne University Press, 60–99.
37. Carey, Hilary M. 1996. *Believing in Australia: A Cultural History of Religions*. St Leonards: Allen and Unwin, 75; Raftery, *Not Part of the Public*, 93; Harris, *One Blood*, 753.
38. Markus, *Governing Savages*, 79; Thomson, Ann. 1988. *NT Dreaming: The Story of the Catholic Church in the Northern Territory*. Darwin: Catholic Education Office, 39; Russo, George. 1980. *Lord Abbot of the Wilderness:*

The Life and Times of Bishop Salvado. Melbourne: The Polding Press, 168–169; Zucker, Margaret. 2005. *From Patrons to Partners And the Separated Children of the Kimberly: A History of the Catholic Church in the Kimberley*, second edition. Fremantle: University of Notre Dame Press, 73.

39. Markus, *Governing Savages*, 84–87; Briscoe, Gordon. 2003. *Counting, Health and Identity: A History of Aboriginal Health and Demography in Western Australia and Queensland 1900–1940*. Australian Capital Territory: Aboriginal Studies Press, 343.
40. Briscoe, *Counting, Health and Identity*, 343; Rowse, Tim. 2017. *Indigenous and Other Australians since 1901*. Sydney: University of New South Wales Press, 167.
41. Francis, Karen. 2001.'Service to the Poor: The Foundations of Community Nursing in England, Ireland and New South Wales.' *International Journal of Nursing Practice* 7 (3), 171; Hogan, *The Irish Missionary Movement*, 55-56; Turner, *Catholics in Australia,* 6.
42. Nelson, Siobhan. 2001. *Say Little, Do Much: Nursing, Nuns and Hospitals in the Nineteenth Century*. University of Pennsylvania Press, 81–89, 96–97.
43. O'Carrigan, Catherine. 1984. 'Australian Catholic Hospitals in the Nineteenth Century.' *Journal of the Australian Catholic History Society* 7, Part 4, 20.
44. O'Brien, Anne. 2005. *God's Willing Workers: Women and Religion in Australia*, Sydney: University of New South Wales Press, 164–165; MacGinley, Rosa. 2005. 'Irish Women Religious and Nineteenth Century Australian Social History.' *Australian Journal of Irish Studies* 5, 141, 143; Turner, *Catholics in Australia*, 171.
45. Edwards, Benjamin. 2008. *Wasps, Tykes and Ecumaniacs: Aspects of Australian Sectarianism 1945–1981*. Brunswick East: Acorn Press, 66; Turner, *Catholics in Australia*, 296–305; Hogan, Michael. 1987. *The Sectarian Strand*. Victoria: Penguin Books, 179.
46. Jacobs, Pat. 2001. 'Exiles in the Wilderness: the pioneer Irish Nuns of St John of God, Beagle Bay and Broome, WA, 1907-1940s.' *Australian Journal of Irish Studies* 1, 107-9; Morris, John. 2001. *The Tiwi: From Isolation to Cultural Change: A History of Encounters between an Island People and Outside Forces*. Darwin: Northern Territory University Press, 116-117.
47. Choo, Christine. 2001. *Mission Girls: Aboriginal Women on Catholic Missions in the Kimberley, Western Australia, 1900–1950*. Crawley: University of Western Australia Press, 60–62.
48. Berndt, Ronald M. and Catherine H. Berndt. 1988. 'Body and Soul. More Than an Episode.' In *Aboriginal Australians and Christian Missions: Ethnographic and Historical Studies*, ed. Tony Swain and Deborah Bird

Rose, Bedford Park: The Australian Association for the Study of Religions, 53.

49. Choo, *Mission Girls*, 60-62, 99.
50. Rawcliffe, *Leprosy in Medieval England*, 1.
51. Blevins, K.E., A.E. Crane, C. Lum, K. Furuta, K. Fox, and A.C. Stone. 2020. 'Evolutionary History of Mycobacterium Leprae in the Pacific Islands.' *Philosophical Transactions of the Royal Society B* 375: 20,190,582, http://dx.doi.org/10.1098/rstb.2019.0582.
52. Thompson, John Ashburton. 1897. *A Contribution to the History of Leprosy*. London: Macmillan, 82, 95; Cumpston, J.H.L. 1928. *Health and Disease in Australia: A History*. Introduced and edited by M.J. Lewis, 1989. Canberra: Australian Government Printing Service, 207-8, 210-213.
53. Thompson, *A Contribution to the History of Leprosy*, 231–233.
54. Kettle, Ellen. 1991. *Health Services in the Northern Territory: A History 1824–1970,* volumes one and two. Darwin: North Australia Research Unit, 27; Hunter, Ernest. 1993. *Aboriginal Health and History: Power and Prejudice in Remote Australia*. Cambridge, New York: Cambridge University Press, 62; Robson, Charmaine. 2020. 'Doctors' Dilemma: Appraising the Rights of New South Wales Leprosy Sufferers, 1890–1950.' *Health and History* 22 (1), 43.
55. On Mud Island: Saunders, Suzanne. 1989. *'A Suitable Island Site': Leprosy in the Northern Territory and the Channel Island Leprosarium 1880–1955*. Darwin: Historical Society of the Northern Territory, 24, 26–27; Kettle, *Health Services*, 28. On Dayman Island: Evans, Raymond. 1969. Charitable institutions of the Queensland Government to 1919. M.A. diss., University of Queensland, 209–10; Robertson, Josephine. 1999. In a State of Corruption: Loathsome Disease and the Body Politic. Ph.D. Diss., University of Queensland, 145–148, 209–210.
56. Watters, Greg. 2012. 'Contaminated by China.' In *Australia's Asia: From Yellow Peril to Asian Century*, ed. David Walker and Agnieszka Sobocinska. Crawley: University of Western Australia Publishing, 31–35.
57. 'The Chinese Cancer.' *The Australian Star*. October 4, 1888, 4; Excerpt from *Worker*, September 21, 1895 in Cronin, Kathryn. 1975. 'The Yellow Agony.' In *Exclusion, Exploitation and Extermination: Race Relations in Colonial Queensland*, ed. Raymond Evans, Kay Saunders and Kathryn Cronin. Sydney: Australia and New Zealand Book Company, 302.
58. Scates, Bruce. 1997. *A New Australia: Citizenship, Radicalism and the First Republic*. Cambridge, Melbourne: Cambridge University Press, 160–161.
59. Saunders, Kay. 1975. 'The Black Scourge.' In Evans, Saunders and Cronin, *Exclusion, Exploitation and Extermination*, 210, 218.
60. Robson, Charmaine. 2020. 'Doctors' Dilemma', 132–138.

61. Edmond, *Leprosy and Empire*, 72–73, 92, 102–103, 107–109, 146–147.
62. Gussow, *Leprosy, Racism & Public Health*, 113.
63. Bashford, Alison. 2004. *Imperial Hygiene: A Critical History of Colonialism, Nationalism and Public Health*. Sydney: Palgrave, 88.
64. Thompson, *A Contribution to the History of Leprosy*, 138–145.
65. *Leprosy Act of 1890*, (NSW); *The Leprosy Act of 1892*, (Qld).
66. O'Brien, Anne. 2008. '"All Creatures of the Living God": Religion and Leprosy in Turn of the Century Queensland.' *History Australia* 5 (2), 40.5–41.5; Evans, Charitable Institutions, 211; Robson, 'Doctors' Dilemma,' 126–149.
67. Rée, Gerald Hugo. 2010. Policing Public Health in Queensland, 1859–1919. PhD Diss., Griffith University, 243–245.
68. Murnane, Sister Ignatius SJG. Interview (interviewer unnamed). Typed transcript. (2.57D), Sisters of St John of God Archives Broome.
69. Correspondence on leprosy and leper colonies. Item ID ITM18270, Queensland State Archives.
70. Rée, Policing Public Health in Queensland, 251.
71. For Mud and Dayman Islands: see note 55; for Friday Island: O'Brien, '"All Creatures of the Living God,"' 40.3–40.4; Bezout Island: Briscoe, *Counting, Health and Identity,* 122–5 and Davidson, W.S. 1978. *Havens of Refuge: A History of Leprosy in Western Australia*. Perth: University of Western Australia Press for the Public Health Department, 15–16.
72. Robertson, In a State of Corruption, 147; Kettle, *Health Services in the Northern Territory*, 28.
73. Cumpston, *Health and Disease in Australia*, 208–209.
74. Davidson, *Havens of Refuge,* 6, 18–25.

CHAPTER 3

The Making of Interwar Leprosy Policy for Indigenous Australians

Between 1923 and 1925, tropical medicine specialist, Cecil Cook, conducted a field survey of leprosy in Australia. The disease, once largely confined to the east, had infiltrated the north of the continent. Mostly, Indigenous people were afflicted but endemicity was present among white Australians in regions of interracial contact. Cook criticised state government control measures and recommended the standardisation of policy under federal government authority. Drawing from international precedents and biomedicine, adapted to local epidemiology, Cook and his colleagues in Australian health bureaucracies determined leprosy policies in the interwar period. As white settlement of the north expanded, a major aim was to protect white Australians from the presumed threat posed by Indigenous people with infectious diseases.

Concomitantly, concern for the health and welfare of remote Indigenous Australians found expression among humanitarians, Indigenous activists, missionaries, and anthropologists, with their agitation for change and giving relief and protection at missions, sometimes subverting leprosy laws. Resultant inquiries did little to lessen harsh leprosy policy. Between 1931 and 1940, leprosaria for Indigenous patients opened in the Northern Territory, north-west Western Australia, and northern Queensland—Channel Island, Derby, and Fantome Island, respectively—supported by funded field surveys and stronger legal powers for examination and detention.

C. Robson, *Missionary Women, Leprosy and Indigenous Australians, 1936–1986*, https://doi.org/10.1007/978-3-031-05796-0_3

Tropical Medicine and Commonwealth Control

The rising influence of the discipline of tropical medicine and the integration of its practitioners in Australian health bureaucracies in the first half of the twentieth century was a major factor in determining leprosy policy for Indigenous patients. Tropical medicine applied the relatively new sciences of bacteriology and parasitology to the treatment of diseases found generally in the warm climate colonies of Europe and the United States, such as in Africa and Asia. It supported imperialistic projects through efforts to protect Europeans in the colonies from disease, but also sought to deliver modern medical treatment to the indigenous inhabitants, with the object of eliminating local outbreaks of disease. Leprosy, although endemic in Norway and Sweden, was classified as a tropical disease: to medical researchers, its near absence in metropolitan centres and growing prevalence in colonial outposts rendered it as exotic as malaria or yellow fever. It was difficult to diagnose, impossible to cure, and the causative bacillus could not be grown in vitro, thus presenting an interesting challenge for medical scientists.

In the 1890s, the first institutions for educating doctors in tropical medicine were established in Western Europe and Britain, including the London School of Tropical Medicine. Among its graduates in the early 1920s were Cecil Cook and Raphael Cilento, both of whom occupied senior positions in Australia's health bureaucracies and would lead the leprosy campaign begun in the interwar years. J.H.L. Cumpston, the first Commonwealth Director-General of Health (1921–1945), also an adherent of tropical medicine, was mentor to both men. The institutes, schools, conferences, and medical journals connected these doctors to international networks with others from Britain, Europe, and the United States, for the sharing of knowledge about tropical disease medicine and its application in the colonial world. In the settler nation of Australia, the effect of the hot northern climate on the long-term survival of the white population in the expanding northern frontiers became a central concern alongside the control of diseases in both white and Indigenous peoples.[1]

Cook's part in Australian leprosy policy can be traced back to his seminal epidemiological study for the Wandsworth Research Scholarship from the London School of Tropical Medicine. Aged twenty-six, he began his two-year field survey of the disease in 1923. He attempted to track and document all present and past cases, his 24,000-mile journey taking him to mainly coastal regions in northern New South Wales, Queensland, the Northern Territory, and northern Western Australia. The resulting report, published in 1927, positioned Cook as the principal authority on leprosy epidemiology and management in Australia. Cumpston endorsed the report as "a complete record of the known facts relating to leprosy in Australia," stating that it offered a "practical possibility of eradicating leprosy completely from Australia."[2]

Cook revisited the questions tackled by Dr John Ashburton Thompson in his 1890s report (see Chapter 2), benefitting from thirty more years of records. He argued that leprosy was spread via person-to-person transmission and that the disease had been unknown in Indigenous populations until European settlement, after which it was introduced to Australia by Chinese and South Sea islander immigrants. Cook's observations led to certain assumptions: Indigenous people did not recognise leprosy when it struck their communities; it typically appeared in places of contact with 'coloured' migrants, and it took a particularly virulent form in them, as with other previously unexposed races.[3] He believed leprosy transmission required "some degree of prolonged and intense exposure between sufferer and susceptible" and occurred either in casual encounters or within the household.[4] Cook argued that indentured workers in Queensland had carried the disease to sugar plantation areas such as Maryborough where he found rises in Indigenous cases. In the Northern Territory, he posited that leprosy spread from the Chinese railway workers in the East Alligator River district to the Indigenous people who then carried it to the Daly and Roper Rivers areas, and on to East Arnhem Land in the 1920s. As for Western Australia, he ascribed the earlier Roebourne outbreak to importation from the Northern Territory.[5] Only later, government leprologist, W.S. Davidson attributed transmission to local Indigenous population to Asian pearling crews who worked the coasts nearby.[6]

Cook categorised means of leprosy transmission as either sexual or household. With the development of rural industries several decades previously, an influx of white men to supply the necessary labour brought them into sexual contact with Indigenous women from whom, Cook assumed, leprosy was passed. Its subsequent transmission by the white male to other members of his household had led to endemicity in the white community.[7] Queensland's experience was a lesson for the Northern Territory and, possibly, Western Australia, where the latest outbreaks in areas of interracial contact had followed increased mining and pastoral activities. By his own admission, leprosy cases in Australia were few but the disease "if left to itself, [it] would in time probably become a menace to successful white settlement."[8]

Cook's recommendations for leprosy control were derived partly from his findings that, despite having the strictest legislation in Australia, Queensland continued to report increasing numbers of cases. He advocated more scrupulous implementation of compulsory notification and isolation of diagnosed cases, and more diligent examinations of contacts. These measures were to apply to all sufferers, regardless of race. However, for leprosy suspects, he advocated home isolation for "responsible" Europeans but leprosarium isolation for Indigenous people because "their careless and irresponsible habits render it impossible to keep him under observation or to submit him to a course of treatment unless he is under restraint."[9]

Other recommendations related to the conditions and treatment within lazarets. Upon inspecting Mud Island in the Northern Territory, and Roebourne and Derby in Western Australia, Cook found that measures to ensure isolation from the healthy were inadequate. Care and treatment of the patients were "neglected or unsatisfactory"—an unjustifiable situation, given the presumed efficacy of current leprosy drugs.[10] He stressed the need for "a skilled attendant having a thorough knowledge of the therapeutic properties of the drugs employed and a complete comprehension of the significance of the various reactions to treatment manifested by individual patients."[11] Cook's preference was for a single leprosarium for all patients from northern Australia, except Queensland (which had Peel Island), securely situated in the Northern Territory under federal government control. The centralised operations would allow for high standard equipment and staff. [12] He saw this model as sound medical and public health practice, and, also, as humane. The leprosarium was to become "to the leper what a sanatorium is to the consumptive, a haven of refuge, rather than a loathsome prison…."[13] People would come forward, rather than evade, the leprosarium, thus ultimately assisting public health goals.[14]

By the time Cook's survey was published, Cilento was based in Queensland as director of the Australian Institute of Tropical Medicine, a division of the Commonwealth Department of Health. Like Cook, Cilento saw poor Indigenous health as an obstacle to settlement by white Australians in the far north. He too believed in federalising health policy to optimise infectious disease control. For Cilento, the far north, encompassing the enormous region abutting the coastal fringes of the continent from the Dampier Archipelago in the north-west to Rockhampton in the north-east, was one vast exotic laboratory but was inconveniently administered from three different centres of government: Western Australia, Queensland, and the Commonwealth, which controlled the Northern Territory Medical Service.[15] The Commonwealth Department of Health, founded in 1921, and headed by John Cumpston, himself an adherent of tropical medicine, was key to mounting the leprosy campaign. Although its formal powers were limited, the Department used indirect means to drive state health policies. The publishing of Cook's *Epidemiology of Leprosy* as a government monograph in 1925 with Cumpston's glowing introduction should not be overlooked as one such strategy. In 1927, Cook, supported by Cumpston, became Chief Medical Officer of the Northern Territory, and simultaneously, the Territory's Chief Protector of Aboriginals and Chief Quarantine Officer, providing the avenue for implementing his leprosy policy proposals. Both he and Cilento were thus able to further health campaigns in the Australian tropics from influential health bureaucracies (Fig. 3.1).

Cumpston's ambition was "of leading this young nation of ours to a paradise of physical perfection."[16] He sought to expand the horizons of his public health brief beyond the limitations imposed by state boundaries. Thus in 1925, the federal government set up the Royal Commission into Health which recommended the formation of the Federal Health Council (FHC).[17] Comprised of representatives of state and Commonwealth Health Departments, this body met regularly to achieve uniform regulations and standards governing infectious disease control and to consider other public health matters.[18] Federal health bureaucrats wielded influence through their access to funding and with their forthright, expert promotion of issues, thereby legitimising Commonwealth authority over the state-controlled area of health.

The first FHC meeting in 1927 resolved to investigate "leprosy and typhus-like diseases in the Commonwealth."[19] Tropical medicine experts, including Cilento, urged further research in this field. But further discussion did not occur until the fifth session in 1931, after Cilento became Director of Tropical Hygiene, and thus representative of the Commonwealth Health Department on the FHC. His paper stated that "leprosy continues its insidious course, and the slow but continual discovery of new cases…represents perhaps the most pressing problem at the moment."[20] Cumpston, drawing on Cook's research, discussed the failure of the existing system in preventing new cases in Queensland

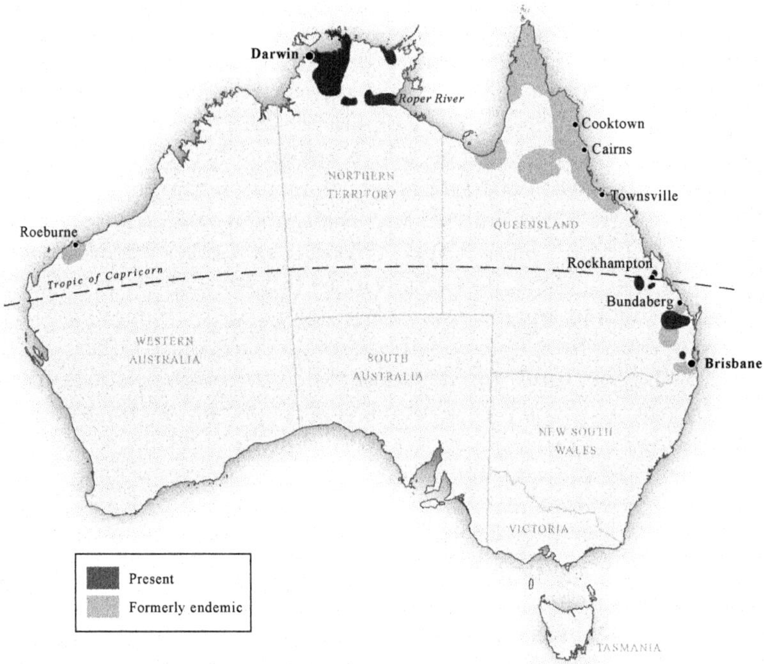

Fig. 3.1 Past and present distribution of leprosy in tropical Australia, based on Report of the Federal Health Council, 5th Session, 1931 (Alan Laver)

and New South Wales. Although only twelve cases had been notified in the previous year, Cumpston proposed a programme for these states and Western Australia to detect hidden cases, meticulously trace the contacts of any newly diagnosed cases, and ensure greater surveillance of patients discharged from lazarets.[21] The FHC formally adopted these recommendations and asked the states to submit all data to the Division of Tropical Hygiene.[22]

The FHC resolution required considerable state resources that were, arguably, disproportionate to the threat posed by the disease to the population. Cumpston admitted that the investigations, especially in Western Australia, would be onerous and expensive, and could prove fruitless.[23]

But such missions, into the deepest reaches of the country, and the accurate documentation of their findings typified the ambitious, military style of tropical medicine. More evidence of this approach can be found in a resolution of the Seventh Session of 1934 following increased notifications in the Western Australian Indigenous population. The FHC asked each state to "provide full legal powers for the periodical examination and any necessary detention of lepers, suspect lepers and contacts."[24] With the growing ratio of Indigenous to European sufferers, control over the former would intensify, and all states would be brought in line with the Northern Territory *Leprosy Ordinance* of 1928 which already contained these provisions.[25]

The Segregation Controversy

From the mid-1920s, some leprologists began arguing for Australia to relax laws enforcing the segregation of leprosy-affected people, arguing that they were inhumane and counterproductive to efforts to eliminate the disease. Impetus for this movement came principally from promising research by British tropical medicine pioneers, Sir Leonard Rogers and Ernest Muir, with an old Indian remedy for leprosy, hydnocarpus oil (known also as *chaulmoogra oil*) and its derivatives in Calcutta. Rogers refined an injectable form to eliminate the severe nausea induced by the traditional oral administration. He and Muir maintained that, under optimum conditions, and if given early in the course of the disease, the infection cleared up and the patient could leave full-time care.[26] By the 1920s, chaulmoogra was the drug of choice for leprosy, internationally, and in Australia.

Rogers argued that under the system of compulsory segregation, people with the early stage of leprosy often avoided treatment, being fearful of lifelong isolation. When debilitating symptoms eventually induced them to come forward, it was too late for the drugs to be effective. During the time they had resisted segregation, they had posed a risk to the healthy people around them, and thus, jeopardised the battle to eradicate the disease.[27]

Certain cases of leprosy, as doctors then knew, were not infectious, as in the early stage of the tuberculoid form, and when the disease spontaneously 'arrested,' that is, reached a state in which no active signs appeared for at least two years. Successful treatment with chaulmoogra oil could also induce this condition. Anti-segregationist doctors opposed isolation of patients in this category. They admitted that there was still uncertainty about when, if ever, arrest would occur, and that a relapse in later years was also a distinct possibility, but with constant supervision by an experienced clinician, any deterioration could be detected and addressed.[28]

In 1930, in the *Medical Journal of Australia (MJA)*, Sir Leonard Rogers denounced Australia's system of compulsory segregation and recommended the policy he had pioneered throughout the British Empire. People with positive bacteriological test results, he argued, should be offered segregation under skilled medical care, and those with negative results, given three-monthly examinations at outpatient facilities. He advocated fresh food and exercise and, preferably, a dry cool climate, the necessary conditions for successful results with chaulmoogra oil.[29] Thousands of patients in India, Africa, and British Guiana had come under his programme, so presumably it could be implemented in Australia for remotely situated Indigenous patients.

To enable his scheme, Rogers trawled the Empire for resources, exploiting the scientific know-how and religious philanthropy of his compatriots. Founding the British Empire Leprosy Relief Association (BELRA) in 1923, he attracted impressive benefactors, the patronage of the Prince of Wales and the advisory services of senior British physicians. He organised specialist leprology training, medication, and surgical supplies, and promoted his treatment principles in existing leprosy facilities, including those run by the Mission to Lepers.[30] In 1933, Toc H volunteers were trained for treating leprosy in Nigeria.[31] His methods were widely reported in medical journals, textbooks, and conferences. Rogers had not found a golden bullet for leprosy but had redefined management strategies, replacing heavy-handed segregation with reliance on sufferers' agency in volunteering for treatment, and optimising their clinical and psychological care.

Prior to Rogers' article, E.H. Molesworth, a dermatologist at Sydney's Royal Prince Alfred Hospital had also taken to the pages of the *MJA* with an impassioned plea on behalf of urban doctors in private practice, describing their dread at diagnosing leprosy in a patient, for he "would rather blow out his brains than face internment."[32] Doctors preferred to avoid this anguish by delaying an early diagnosis, based on clinical signs, until a bacteriological examination proved positive, thus deferring vital medical treatment. Patients also evaded medical attention until their condition worsened. Echoing Rogers and Muir, Molesworth expounded on the deleterious effect of this avoidance of treatment on the patient's prognosis and eradication of the disease. He advocated voluntary admission to a hospital, rather than a lazaret, and superior medical treatment.[33]

But Molesworth's concerns were not for the welfare of the Indigenous leprosy sufferer. He had "seen the tragedy in a man's eyes and heard the despair in an educated European's voice…at being told that he must go to the lazaret…"[34] His sympathies lay with middle- to upper-class white men, people like himself. Here he departed from Rogers, whose call for modifying isolation was prompted by his work among non-European colonised people. Indigenous people fell so far outside Molesworth's consideration that he opposed their compulsory segregation only because "the majority of aboriginal lepers cannot be found, caught nor kept," and declared that their imminent extinction would ultimately make such efforts redundant.[35] Although Cumpston did not agree, he shared Molesworth's moral dilemma about the better off European diagnosed with leprosy:

> For Chinese, Kanakas and Aborigines, isolation under the strictest control is obviously all that can be considered. For Europeans who are indigent or feeble-minded a similar control is necessary. The remainder of the Europeans present the great problem of leprosy administration.[36]

Conflated with the poor, non-white and mentally defective, Indigenous people presented no such quandary: officials could justify stripping whatever freedoms remained from those already disenfranchised. Similarly, they rationalised the permanent isolation of Indigenous people from their homes by pointing out the inadequate nutrition, health services, and accommodation in home communities. To return to these areas risked relapse and further leprosy transmission.[37]

Given the inadequate services for Indigenous communities, Rogers' suggested alternative to the leprosarium—treatment stations close to leprosy outbreaks—would always prove challenging for Australian governments.[38] As Cook showed, leprosy occurred in widely scattered communities across vast distances. Even with government funding, qualified health personnel and infrastructure would be difficult to obtain. Among missionaries, the most likely to agree to such work, these qualifications were rare. Yet, missionaries daily confronted Indigenous ill-health, including leprosy, as will be discussed.

Humanitarians and Missionaries

While the threat of leprosy to the white population was a crucial matter for health administrators, a concomitant, significant wave of concern for Indigenous people with the disease, emerged in the interwar period by those with largely humanitarian or religious motives. It took two distinctive forms: a predominantly urban-based activism demanding policy change with respect to Indigenous health and welfare generally, and the day-to-day efforts by missionaries and others to address shortfalls in government services to Indigenous people. The latter sometimes entailed active resistance to official policy.

In October 1927, scientists, clergymen, female philanthropists, and Indigenous activists presented a petition to Federal parliament warning that the Indigenous race was dying out and proposing the establishment of a separate Indigenous state for their protection and social "advancement."[39] Governments, the petition claimed, were responsible, as they had failed to prevent the "blighting influence of immoral Europeans": violence, introduced diseases, and the deprivation of food sources.[40] Only a few Europeans would be permitted in the "model state," including missionary administrators, until transition to self-government, and there would be "rigorous medical control and treatment of contagious diseases."[41]

The petition was one of several attempts to alert the nation to the sub-standard living conditions and treatment of Indigenous peoples. The previous May, a deputation by missionaries and anthropologists to federal Parliament had requested a royal commission.[42] The lobbying continued, drawing support from welfare organisations, including the newly formed Aborigines Protection League, print media coverage, and sympathetic federal politicians. Finally, in 1928, the Commonwealth government announced an investigation into the "present status and conditions of aboriginals and half-castes in Central Australia and North Australia."[43] The Queensland Protector of Aborigines, J.W. Bleakley, was temporarily relieved of his duties to carry out the inquiry.

Bleakley painted a grim picture of Indigenous health among the inhabitants of Central and North Australia, and criticised current government arrangements for their care. He witnessed cases of leprosy on the eastern coast of the Northern Territory and others held in primitive conditions of isolation at Roper River and Groote Eylandt missions, noting, "It is possible that the mission authorities, if assisted financially, could secure the services of a trained medical missionary for work in this area."[44] Of Mud Island Lazaret he was also highly critical, condemning the poor accommodation and the absence of nursing care. What little care was given was supplied by a patient of mixed descent under instruction from the Health Department. Bleakley thought missionaries were more appropriate carers than government officers since they worked from "missionary and not mercenary motives," and he recommended increased funding for missions and the establishment of more mission stations.[45] He further suggested that the need for medical relief was so urgent and so widespread that the wives of male missionaries—whom he termed "missionary mothers"—should act as nurses in strategically located "relief camps."[46]

After the report's release, it was discussed at a meeting of mission representatives, pastoralists, and government officials. Several missionaries proposed the transfer of Indigenous affairs from state to federal control, since the states had been miserly and uncooperative.[47] Unsurprisingly, they supported Bleakley's suggestion for their own stronger involvement in the administration of Indigenous institutions, but they desperately required more government support. Church of England missionaries explained that they lacked the skills to diagnose and treat leprosy and other serious diseases at their missions, one claiming that a visit by a doctor had been promised four years previously but had still not occurred.[48]

Cook, whose views were sought, advised against greater participation by missionaries, with special aversion to Bleakley's 'missionary mothers.' "The substitution of motherly women for qualified medical practitioners and double certificated nurses is a recommendation concerning which the least said the better."[49] Cook had little tolerance for assigning underqualified personnel to healthcare roles.

In 1930, Federal Minister, Arthur Blakeley, formally rejected the health reforms suggested in Bleakley's report. He almost implied that the investigation had been unnecessary, and that the groundswell of protest had been based on fiction:

> No action is necessary in connection with Mr. Bleakley's recommendations that regular medical inspection should be provided for bush blacks, that Aboriginal clinics should be provided where medical assistance is available, also on mission stations, that first aid medical guides and medicine chests should be provided at all relief stations, that blankets and clothing

> should be supplied to destitutes in semi-civilised camps, and that regular inspections of institutions and district operations should be carried out. Action along the lines suggested has been taken by the Administration for a number of years.[50]

Bleakley's report failed to spur the federal government into prompt and humane measures for Indigenous health and welfare, ranking it with its state counterparts of whom it had been so critical.

In this period, missionaries sometimes violated public health laws by refusing to notify authorities of those in their care with leprosy. Missionaries believed they offered better care, spiritually and physically, than at government lazarets, and they saw the people as their responsibility and members of their mission communities. Some had nursing personnel, such as at Groote Eylandt in the Northern Territory and Beagle Bay in north-west Western Australia. The missionaries at Oenpelli in the Northern Territory were remembered for their kindness to those with leprosy "who came in from the bush."[51] One missionary explained, "They would only stay on condition that I did not send them to Darwin."[52] In 1927, the Anglican Bishop of Carpentaria ordered superintendents of missions under his authority not to send patients to Mud Island, as it was devoid of both physical and spiritual care.[53] However, some missions were supplied with appropriate medication and treatment advice in the expectation they would provide services to leprosy patients until accommodation at a lazaret could be found.[54]

Missionaries also pressed the case for better treatment of the Indigenous leprosy-affected through letters to the press or their respective governments.[55] Ministers of various denominations who asked permission to open their own leprosaria were universally turned down. In August 1930, Otto Raible, Catholic Vicar Apostolic for Broome, applied to the West Australian government to open a lazaret at Swan Point near the Lombadina Mission. Patients would be segregated from mission residents and come under the direct charge of the religious. Food and transport would be supplied by the mission. The lazaret would have the services of a mission doctor and be managed by two nurses from the Sisters of St John of God trained in leprosy nursing care. As Raible indicated, superior care to that at Cossack would be offered and the patients, most being from the Kimberley, would be closer to their homes. His offer was declined. The government was satisfied with relying on missionaries as a stopgap, but did not wish to relinquish full control over leprosy patients, despite the financial advantage.[56]

Indigenous Ideas About Leprosy

Whether missionary, doctor, or health official, the isolation of the leprosy sufferer was a common aim of white authorities, based on science, and spiritual and physical welfare considerations. Based on research undertaken in Arnhem Land, it is clear that Indigenous people had different understandings of leprosy and how to deal with it. To make sense of a new and debilitating physical affliction that infiltrated communities from the early twentieth century, they incorporated ideas about causation, prognosis, and treatments into existing traditional law. Leprosy in the Yolngu language is *borrpoi*. It is the same word for the marring and degeneration of body tissue that is believed to occur as retribution for violations of traditional customs. The word *borrpoi* is also the term for payback. Various means are used by spirits or sorcerers to enact payback, including drawing pictures of a person on trees and rubbing poison into them, piercing a person's footprints or burning then concealing their soiled clothing, leading to physical symptoms such as sores and swellings, then death.[57]

Indigenous people have not usually attributed leprosy to person-to-person transmission, nor does their culture carry the Western stigma associated with it, therefore they have not been fearful of others with the disease. Their reaction has been not to turn the afflicted away but to treat them "with love and inclusion" and provide them what care they could.[58] Karen Hughes shows evidence of this care in her study of nurse Ruth Heathcock who covertly attended to the surgical and medical needs of leprosy sufferers hidden in the bush, in fear of missions and the lazaret. After some experience of leprosy, Indigenous people learnt to identify it and became "aware of symptoms presaging deformity or isolation"; they became adept at evading patrols by police and doctors.[59] As shown in the next section, these reactions of Indigenous people to leprosy partly shaped the actions of Australian health authorities, in their dogged campaigns to locate sufferers and to remove them to institutions remote from country.

The Leprosaria for Indigenous People

Channel Island Leprosarium

In 1931, the Commonwealth Health Department opened the promised new 'central leprosarium' on Channel Island in the Northern Territory, about ten kilometres by sea from Darwin, reflecting Chief Medical Officer Cook's preference for strict segregation and the centralisation of control. Patients were drawn from the Northern Territory and from the region in Western Australia north of the 28th degree of south latitude, under an agreement by the respective governments.[60] The passage of the *Leprosy Ordinance 1928* expanded powers for examining and isolating leprosy suspects, as Cook had recommended and his preference for an island location was satisfied. Since most patients were Indigenous, the risk that they would abscond was thought to be high, for "the native is deeply attached to the society of his own tribe and tends to become despondent or attempt escape when confined to a strange country."[61] They could only be successfully confined on the mainland "with walls of a very substantial construction" and, according to Chief Health Officer, Henry Leighton-Jones in 1926, this would be unnecessarily inhumane in depriving them totally of the freedom they had left behind[62] (Fig. 3.2).

As Cook himself had acknowledged, an island leprosarium limited doctors' access to the patients and therefore compromised his aim for up-to-the-minute medical treatment.[63] Few doctors would have been willing to reside on the lonely and primitive Channel Island. Medical visits had to be fitted into an overloaded, difficult schedule, subject to the often adverse weather conditions of Darwin Harbour.[64] Not only was the supervision of patients' treatment hampered, but so too was the availability of emergency medical attention.

Even more important therefore was Cook's insistence on installing resident qualified nursing staff. He declined to engage one married couple as carers as neither had professional nurse training.[65] Mrs. Jenkinson, the first matron, was a registered nurse who had received specialist leprosy training at Peel Island leprosarium before beginning at Channel Island in 1931.[66] A hospital was built for inmates requiring inpatient care and treatment began with the latest therapy, chaulmoogra oil. Leprosy nursing also involved managing pain, bandaging, and cleaning sores, tending to the dying, and assisting in childbirth. On Mud Island, any such tasks could only have been carried out by the residents.

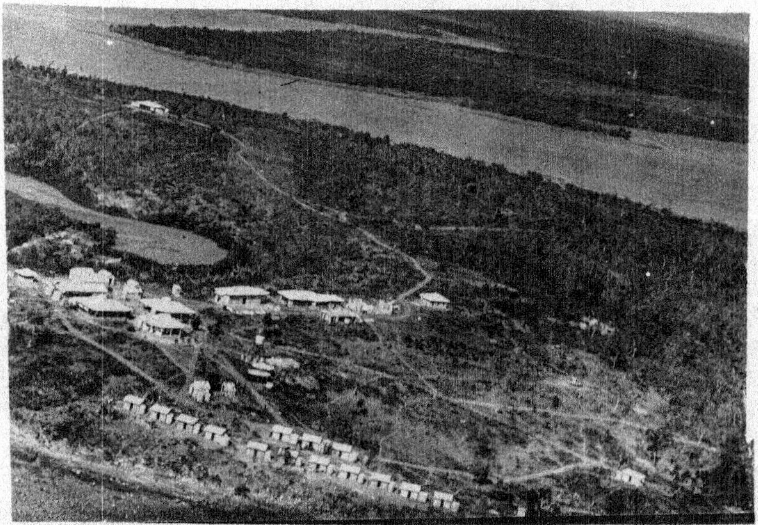

Fig. 3.2 Aerial view of Channel Island Leprosarium 1940 (By Alexander Murray. Library and Archives NT)

The matron's husband was employed as curator, or superintendent, in a trend that would continue over the ensuing decade, as one couple left, and another replaced them. Several curators had previously worked in positions of authority over Indigenous people as Protectors of Aboriginals, police, or institutional superintendents.[67] Their most vital role in the leprosarium was controlling the behaviour of the male patients. Violence and sexual advances to the female patients were expected consequences of forcibly detaining and sexually segregating strong young men. Women of mixed descent were seen to need particular protection as, until the presence of European staff could be guaranteed, they were isolated at Darwin hospital rather than Mud Island.[68] Presumably, the purity of Indigenous women did not hold the same value for state authorities.

The curator allocated jobs to the fitter male patients and took charge of supplies. To some extent, the curator and matron adopted parental roles—the curator in the conventional father's role of disciplinarian, able to do some manual labour and perhaps instruct male patients in some of the skills conventionally undertaken by European men, and the matron in the mother's roles of nurse and nurturer. The previous experience of Elsie and Jack Jones as managers of a home for mixed descent children would have been valuable in fostering a settlement-style community within the leprosarium where they had charge from 1937 until 1942.

But by the outbreak of World War II, Channel Island leprosarium had slipped considerably from Cook's ideal. The island had insufficient water to support the cultivation of fruit and vegetables, food deemed essential for patients' health. Water for cooking and washing had to be shipped from the mainland. As patient numbers rose, from an initial 50 to 129 by 1939, Matron Jones could not cope with the nursing and began training girls of mixed descent as unpaid nursing aides. Medical records were not kept, and doctors visited infrequently. The patients' health did not seem to improve under these conditions, for at least 60 people died in this period.[69]

Perhaps, the most devastating aspect of the 'central leprosarium' was the removal of people from their homes. Some, from the bush, were abruptly swept up in 'leper' patrols, clapped in neck chains and forced to walk for miles. For Western Australians, this ordeal was followed by detention at a temporary holding place until they were again set in chains, picked up by lugger, and taken the 1000 km to Darwin.[70] These voyages, made in wild weather and on unseaworthy vessels, were notorious for inflicting "unspeakable discomfort" on their passengers, in the words of one captain.[71] The extent to which this experience, combined with the pain of leaving family and country, contributed to a declining state of health can never be measured.

Derby Leprosarium

Sending Western Australian patients to the Northern Territory did little to remove the spectre of a dangerous and unmanaged infectious disease in the north-west by the early 1930s. As Channel Island became crowded and with the Cossack lazaret demolished, new cases, mainly from the Western Kimberley, accumulated. Most were placed in the Derby Native Hospital grounds under the charge of Cossack's former curator and matron, Effie and Frank Luyer. A small number were isolated in shacks at the Beagle Bay Mission, waiting for the next ship bound for Darwin, sometimes for periods as long as eighteen months. The Western Australia Public Health Department provided subsidies to the personnel at both lazarets for the maintenance of the patients and their leprosy medication.[72]

Both parties in charge of these ad hoc lazarets appeared to work conscientiously and to the best of their abilities under extraordinarily difficult circumstances. Nurse Luyer and some of the SSJG Sisters were trained nurses. In failing to ensure that professional medical care and judgement were available to those detained, however, the state government was deeply negligent. At the mission, this was eventually remedied in 1935 by the appointment of two doctors trained in tropical medicine from Germany.[73]

At Derby, leprosy work was only a small part of the aged District Medical Officer's hefty workload, much of which took him out of town for long periods, leaving the Luyers to diagnose and treat patients. Nurse Luyer relied on correspondence with the Commissioner of Public Health, Western Australia (CPH), Everitt Atkinson, for treatment advice. For advanced cases, for which she held no hope, she had her own device: "I make up a large bottle of medicine, composed of a little Epsom salts and cochineal to make it a pretty colour, this they get each day and they think they are getting better, it keeps them contented."[74] Albert Davis, Medical Officer for the Department of Aborigines, complained that treatment was not based "upon scientific lines [therefore] they do not altogether react to the comfort of the patient nor are they always conducive to safe treatment."[75] Some people were erroneously diagnosed and unnecessarily confined for years after which, on reexamination, they were discharged as unproven cases. The personal impact on those people can only be imagined. The errors artificially inflated public health statistics and swelled numbers in the small Derby lazaret to almost fifty people in 1934.[76] Pressure came to bear on the state government from the Derby general public, the press, and the municipal authorities who demanded the removal of the 'lepers' from the proximity of town and the provision of appropriate care.[77]

The leprosy problem was again highlighted in 1934 when the Western Australian government appointed a Royal Commission to "investigate, report and advise upon matters in relation to the condition and treatment of Aborigines" under Magistrate Henry Moseley. Adverse publicity of these issues nationally and overseas had prompted the inquiry.[78] Special reference was to be made, among other items, to "disease amongst aboriginals, and measures for their treatment." After investigating leprosy in the Kimberley, Moseley declared it a priority, and issued an interim report before the completion of the inquiry.[79] He highlighted the lax security at the Derby lazaret, which allowed contact between the inmates and the public, although "it is possible that medical opinion is divided as to the infectivity of leprosy."[80] He relied on Cook's submission stressing the need for stricter isolation, "and I am not inclined to reject his opinion until someone of greater experience in the same branch of the medical profession satisfies me that he is in error."[81]

Moseley condemned the transfer of patients to Channel Island, although this idea had originally been Cook's: "In spite of the utter discomfort and wretchedness obtaining under the present system, the only request I had from the patients was that they should not be sent to Darwin."[82] The policy, he maintained, was counterproductive since the fear of being sent so far from country induced many to abscond. In conclusion, Moseley recommended a thorough inspection of the north-west region for leprosy, abandonment of the Darwin policy, and the erection of a state leprosarium, possibly on Sunday Island. There the residents could reside in huts, go fishing, and be locked in at night to prevent their escape.[83]

Moseley's proposal aimed at balancing the predicament of leprosy sufferers, with whom he evidently sympathised, with the alleged public health crisis. As with the Bleakley inquiry, public lobbying for improved Indigenous welfare had prompted this investigation. Whether sufferers would be better off as a result is difficult to assess, but, by following Cook's advice, as had been done with Bleakley's report, leprosarium policy in north-west Western Australia would be similar to that in the Northern Territory.

Moseley's recommendations were adopted, but, as Sunday Island was too remote for regular medical visitation, the leprosarium was built about ten miles from the town of Derby near the mudflats of the King Sound coast.[84] Cilento, whose recommendations had been sought by the Public Health Commissioner, had stressed permanent isolation for Indigenous leprosy sufferers well away from endemic areas—which, of course, were often their home regions. He advised that "Every aboriginal leper should be removed and should never return".[85]

The Western Australian government baulked at paying fully for construction, arguing that "the care of the aborigines is really a national question" and too costly for a state with a high proportion of Indigenous compared with white people. After the federal government was approached for financial assistance, the Prime Minister addressed Cabinet:

> It can hardly be denied that in some degree the safety of Australia depends upon the development of the north. This in turn depends upon the condition of public health safety of that region, and in order to ensure such public health safety... a leper station for aborigines ... is definitely necessary.[86]

Again, leprosy control was framed as necessary for white settlement. Cabinet approved half the construction cost (£5000) but not maintenance costs.[87] In 1937, the National Health and Medical Research Council (NHMRC), the successor of the FHC, funded a travelling medical officer for a leprosy survey of the Kimberley. The leprosarium was completed in December 1936 and ninety patients were admitted early the next year.[88]

Regarding staff, Davis advised employing "a professional man" to provide "the best possible treatment."[89] Aware that such personnel was difficult to obtain "in Australia, for the prejudice is too great," he suggested that the Health Department appoint a medical missionary through BELRA, whom Nurse Luyer could assist.[90] Davis' advice was not followed and when the leprosarium opened, the Luyers were once again in charge.

Fantome Island Leprosarium

The third institution opened in 1940 on Fantome Island in northern Queensland, near the port of Townsville. It was exclusively for 'coloured' (a term mainly denoting Aboriginal and Torres Strait Islander peoples and Pacific Islanders) patients, many of whom had been detained at Peel Island leprosarium near Brisbane, with white patients until the change in policy to racially segregated institutions. Rosalind Kidd argues that Bleakley saw it as a means of restoring his authority over Indigenous patients who, as Peel Island inmates, were under Health Department control.[91] Accessed via the Indigenous 'island penitentiary,' Palm Island, and sharing its location with a venereal diseases lock hospital for Indigenous people, Fantome Island leprosarium was linked to a system of offshore removal, designed, ironically, to protect the white mainland population from the casualties of European settlement—the maladjusted, disorderly, and diseased.

The leprosarium was in effect a joint venture of the state and Commonwealth Health Departments, the culmination of much planning, lobbying, and research, spearheaded by Cilento after becoming Queensland Director-General of Health in 1935. This position, together with his influence at the FHC and the NHMRC, secured Commonwealth and state government support for his ambition of tackling diseases of Indigenous people in northern Queensland. His Queensland appointment also facilitated the implementation of Commonwealth Health Department policies in the state-controlled domains of health and Indigenous affairs.[92]

Kidd's research documents Cilento's continual frustration at the negligence of Queensland's Indigenous affairs bureaucracies regarding conditions at settlements and missions. Insufficient funding and supervision meant that hygiene, diet, and medical and nursing care were abysmally inadequate. According to Cilento, this environment fostered the spread of infectious diseases and "continue[s] to threaten the survival of the race and to fill the Lazaret."[93]

In June 1937, Cilento's application to the NHMRC for a grant for leprosy investigation in northern Queensland was approved.[94] Meanwhile, the corresponding application by the Western Australia Commissioner of Public Health was under consideration. The Council's support was due to its concern at the "tendency of leprosy to spread in two of the states amongst aborigines and to a lesser but definite extent amongst whites."[95] In the period 1926–1930, twenty-eight people were admitted to the Peel Island leprosarium compared with sixty-two in the following five-year period.[96] Cilento mentioned "the increased number of coloured lepers detected" in his grant application as justifying further inquiry.[97] Although "there has been no outstanding increase" since leprosy was first notified in Queensland fifty years previously, and it had been endemic in Queensland Europeans for many years, he suspected greater numbers of Indigenous people were infected, beyond the reach of diagnosticians and with the potential for wider dissemination throughout Indigenous and European populations.[98] To these ends, Cilento intensified a field study already begun at the Mona Mona Mission, home of a disproportionate number of closely related patients recently admitted to Peel Island, and conducted research at Palm Island and Yarrabah.

Developments supporting this venture followed in rapid succession. New provisions under Section 51 of the Queensland Health Act in 1937 broadened the powers of the Queensland Director-General of Health, allowing medical examinations of suspects and their contacts without their consent.[99] The following year, Cilento received another Commonwealth grant, this time to establish a research station in the Palm Island group, the objectives of which were specified by the NHMRC:

a. Establishing more precisely than is known at present the course of leprosy in aboriginal sufferers and the factors in the spread of leprosy;
b. Improving the treatment of leprosy;
c. Defining humane but efficient measures for the control of leprosy, especially among aborigines. The peculiar difficulties presented by the conditions under which aborigines live have not yet been adequately met by present measures of control.[100]

Leprosy Investigation Officer, Graham Croll, left for North Queensland in early 1939 "to investigate in detail all collections of aboriginals above the 20th degree of South Latitude."[101] The initial survey, covering settlements south of Cairns—Woorabinda, Palm and Fantome Islands, and Yarrabah—yielded very few bacteriologically proven cases of leprosy except for Palm Island where twenty-five were diagnosed and another twenty-seven showed clinical signs only.[102] No active cases were found at all in the next part of the investigation which took Croll to the cattle stations and settlements in the Cape York Peninsula.[103]

The state government decided to open a leprosarium close to the proposed research station in the Palm Island group to accommodate leprosy-affected people detected in the investigations. All Indigenous patients from Peel Island would also be admitted, leaving that leprosarium for Europeans only. Following a visit to Palm Island in March 1939 by Cilento and Bleakley, a site was chosen for the leprosarium and research laboratory at the northern extremity of Fantome Island, 70 km across the sea.

Notes

1. Neill, Deborah. 2012. *Networks in Tropical Medicine: Internationalism, Colonialism, and the Rise of a Medical Specialty, 1890–1930*. Palo Alto: Stanford University Press, 6–7, 15.
2. Cumpston, J.H.L. 1927. 'Preface.' In Cecil Cook, *The Epidemiology of Leprosy in Australia: Being the Report of an Investigation in Australia During the Years 1923–1925 Under the Terms of the Wandsworth*

Research Scholarship of the London School of Tropical Medicine. Canberra: Department of Health.
3. Cook, *Epidemiology*, 260–261.
4. Ibid., 89, 290.
5. Ibid., 40–43, 63–64, 264, 297.
6. Davidson, W.S. 1978. *Havens of Refuge: A History of Leprosy in Western Australia*. Nedlands: University of Western Australia Press, 12–14.
7. Cook, *Epidemiology*, 20.
8. Ibid., 291.
9. Ibid., 298. A "suspect" showed clinical signs of leprosy but yielded negative bacteriological test results.
10. Ibid.
11. Cook, *Epidemiology*, 291.
12. Ibid., 296.
13. Cook, Cecil. 1924. 'Leprosy in Australia' (Correspondence). *Medical Journal of Australia* (*MJA*). September 1, 337.
14. Cook, *Epidemiology*, 298–299.
15. Cilento, R.W. 1931. 'Review of the Position of Tropical Medicine and Hygiene in Australia.' Appendix No. II, Report of the Federal Health Council, Fifth Session, 24–25 March, 20.
16. Roe, Michael. 2006. 'Cumpston, John Howard Lidgett (1880–1954).' In *Australian Dictionary of Biography*, National Centre of Biography, Australian National University, http://adb.anu.edu.au/biography/cumpston-john-howard-lidgett-5846/text9935. Accessed 25 November 2009.
17. Royal Commission on Health. 1926. *Report of the Royal Commission on Health: Together with Appendices*. Victoria: Government of the Commonwealth of Australia, 18.
18. *Commonwealth of Australia Gazette*, 114, November 23, 1926 (A1928, 362/3), National Archives of Australia.
19. 'Federal Health Council.' *The West Australian*, February 8, 1927, 8.
20. Cilento, 'Review of the Position of Tropical Medicine and Hygiene in Australia.'
21. Cumpston, J.H.L. 1931. 'Review of the Administrative Control of Leprosy.' Appendix No. III, Report of the Federal Health Council, Fifth Session, 24–25 March, 34–35.
22. Report of the Federal Health Council, Resolution 17, Fifth Session, 4.
23. Cumpston, 'Review of the Administrative Control of Leprosy.'
24. Cumpston to Secretary, Dept. of the Interior, August 1, 1934 (A659, 1939/1/10643), NAA.
25. *Leprosy Ordinance 1928* (NT).
26. Rogers, Sir Leonard. 1930. 'When will Australia adopt Modern Prophylactic Measures Against Leprosy?' *MJA*. October 1, 525.

27. Ibid., 525.
28. Rogers, Leonard and Ernest. Muir. 1946. *Leprosy*, third edition. Baltimore: The Williams and Wilkins Co., 204–205, 253–254.
29. Ibid., 246–254, 527.
30. Rogers, Sir Leonard. 1950. *Happy Toil: Fifty-Five Years of Tropical Medicine*. London: Muller, 202–204; 'The Economic Aspect of Leprosy.' *The British Medical Journal*, May 6, 1933, 793–794.
31. Rogers, *Happy Toil*, 206.
32. Molesworth, E.H. 1926. 'The Leprosy Problem.' *MJA*, September 1, 378.
33. Ibid., 369, 376.
34. Ibid., 378.
35. Molesworth, E.H. 1927. 'Leprosy' (Correspondence). *MJA*, March 12, 389–390.
36. Cumpston, J.H.L. 1928. *Health and Disease in Australia: A History*. Introduced and edited by M.J. Lewis. Canberra: Australian Government Printing Service, 1989, 217.
37. Johnson, D.W. 1938. 'Report on Peel Island Lazaret for 1937–38.' In Queensland Department of Health and Home Affairs, *Annual Report on the Health & Medical Services of the State of Queensland for the year 1937–1938*. Brisbane: The State, 18; Cilento to Cumpston. July 31, 1934 (A1928, 635/34), NAA.
38. Saunders, Suzanne, 1989. *'A Suitable Island Site': Leprosy in the Northern Territory and the Channel Island Leprosarium 1880–1955*. Darwin: Historical Society of the Northern Territory, 10.
39. Roe, Michael 1986. 'A Model Aboriginal State.' *Aboriginal History*, 10, 40–46.
40. *Petition for A Model Aboriginal State* cited in Roe, 'A Model Aboriginal State,' 41–42; 'Aboriginals.' *Canberra Times*, October 18, 1927, 4.
41. *Petition for A Model Aboriginal State*, 41.
42. 'Condition of Aborigines.' *The Argus*, May 4, 1927, 13.
43. Bleakley, J.W. 1929. 'Aboriginals and Half-Castes of Central Australia and North Australia: Report.' Melbourne: Government Printer.
44. Ibid., 33.
45. Ibid., 19, 24–25.
46. Ibid., 11.
47. 'Report of Debates of the Conference of Representatives of Mission, Societies and Associations interested in the Welfare of Aboriginals to consider the Report and Recommendations submitted to the Commonwealth Government by J.W. Bleakley Esq. convened by the Minister for Home Affairs and held at Masonic Hall, Collins St. Melbourne, 12 April 1929,' 16–17 (A659, 1943/1/1451 Part 1), NAA.
48. Ibid., 239.

49. Cook to Government Resident, June 11, 1929 (A431, 1946/3026), NAA.
50. Publicity Officer, Prime Minister's Department. 'Press Release. Half-Caste Problem. Government's Decision.' July 8, 1930. A659, 1943/1/1451 Part 10, NAA.
51. Constance Bush quoted in Harris, John. 1990. *One Blood: Two Hundred Years of Aboriginal Encounter with Christianity: A Story of Hope*. Sutherland: Albatross Books, 728.
52. Superintendent, Oenpelli Mission to Minister for Home and Territories, c. March 1928 (A431 1950/3597), NAA.
53. Bishop of Carpentaria. 1927. Letter to the Editor, *The Argus*, May 28, 34.
54. Briscoe, Gordon. 2003. *Counting, Health, and Identity: A History of Aboriginal Health and Demography in Western Australia and Queensland 1900-1940*. Canberra: Aboriginal Studies Press, 170.
55. Eddy, W.J. 1928. 'Lepers May Be Increased By Wrong Methods.' *Northern Standard*, October 26, 3; Needham, J.S. 1928. 'The Aborigines: Callous Treatment in the North.' *Sydney Morning Herald*, September 19, 16; John Burton to Secretary, Home and Territories Department, October 26, 1928 (A431 1950/3597), NAA.
56. Davidson, *Havens of Refuge*, 37–38.
57. Cawte, John. 2001. *Healers of Arnhem Land*. Marleston: J.B. Books, 61; Reid, J.C. and D. Mununggurr. 1977. 'We Are Losing our Brothers: Sorcery and Alcohol in an Aboriginal Community.' *MJA*, November 26, 2–3.
58. Hughes, Karen. 2005. '"Same Bodies, Different Skin": Ruth Heathcock.' In *Uncommon Ground: White Women in Aboriginal History*, ed. Anna Cole, Victoria Haskins, and Fiona Paisley. Canberra: Aboriginal Studies Press, 83–106.
59. *Leprosy in Northern Territory Aborigines*. Darwin: Northern Territory Medical Service, 1968, 7–8; Saunders, Suzanne.1990. 'Isolation: The Development of Leprosy Prophylaxis in Australia.' *Aboriginal History* 14, 171.
60. Premier, Western Australia to Prime Minister, 1 September 1927 (A461, G347/1/10 Part 1), NAA.
61. Cook, Cecil. 1924. 'Report of Dr Cecil Cook as a result of his investigations into the conditions in the North-West of Western Australia,' Part IV Granuloma Venereum, 3 (PHD, 1923/1765; SROWA, Cons 1003).
62. Leighton-Jones, H. to Acting Administrator, Northern Territory Government, May 29, 1926 (A431, 1950/3597), NAA.
63. 'Report of Dr Cecil Cook,' Part III Derby Lazaret, 5.
64. Saunders, Suzanne. 1986."A Suitable Island Site": Leprosy in the Northern Territory and the Channel Island Leprosarium 1880–1955. B.Arts Diss., Murdoch University, 121.

65. Kettle, Ellen, 1991. *Health Services in the Northern Territory: A History 1824–1970*, volume one. Darwin: North Australia Research Unit, 109.
66. Parliament of the Commonwealth of Australia. 1932. *Report on the Administration of the Northern Territory for the Year Ended 30th June 1931*. Canberra: Government of the Commonwealth of Australia, 22.
67. Examples of temporary and permanent superintendents at Channel Island are: Ted Heathcock and Vic Hall, both policemen and the Joneses, formerly in charge of the children's home, the Bungalow.
68. *Report on the Administration of the Northern Territory for the year ended 30th June 1931*, 22.
69. Kettle, *Health Services*, 109–110; Saunders, '*A Suitable Island Site*' (1989), 103, 107, 109–114, 132–133.
70. Puertollano, Theresa. 1992. Interview with Christine Choo. Sound Recording (OH2695/34), State Library of Western Australia; see also Jebb, Mary Anne. 2002. *Blood, Sweat and Welfare: A History of White Bosses and Aboriginal Pastoral Workers*. Crawley: University of Western Australia Press, 139–143.
71. 'Leper Transport.' *West Australian*, July 7, 1934, 17.
72. Davidson, *Havens of Refuge*, 37–40, 57–58; 'Lepers in the North.' *The West Australian*, June 25, 1934, 7.
73. Holmes, J.J. 'Leprosy and the Treatment of Aborigines,' June 1, 1936 (Cons 1003, PHD, 1935/0732), State Records Office Western Australia (SROWA).
74. Luyer to Atkinson, November 24, 1933 (Cons 1003, PHD, 1933/0907), SROWA; other correspondence at 1935/0732 & 1933/0907, SROWA.
75. Davis to Atkinson, September 9, 1936 (Cons 1003, PHD, 1935/0732), SROWA.
76. Davis, Albert. 1938. 'Health.' In Western Australia Department of Native Affairs. *Annual Report of the Commissioner of Native Affairs for the Year Ending 30 June 1937*. Perth: Government Printer, 10; Davis to Atkinson, July 13, 1937 (Cons 1003, PHD, 1935/0251), SROWA.
77. Secretary, West Kimberley Road Board to A.A. Coverley, December 21, 1933 (Cons 1003, PHD, 1933/0907), SROWA; 'Lepers in the North,' 7.
78. Haebich, Anna. 1988. *For Their Own Good: Aborigines and Government in the Southwest of Western Australia 1900–1940*. Crawley: University of Western Australia Press, 322–328.
79. Moseley, H.D. 1935. *Report of the Royal Commissioner Appointed to Investigate, Report, and Advise Upon Matters in Relation to the Condition and Treatment of Aborigines*. Perth: Government. Printer, 10.
80. Ibid. 11.
81. Ibid.

82. Ibid.
83. Ibid.
84. Atkinson, Everitt. Memo, June 1935 (Cons. 1003, 1935–0251), SROWA.
85. Cilento to Cumpston, July 31, 1934 (A1928, 635/34), NAA.
86. Lyons, Joseph to Cabinet, November 20, 1935 (A1928, 635/43 SECTION 1), NAA.
87. Department of the Prime Minister to Premier of Western Australia. December 9, 1935 (Cons. 1003, 1935–0251), SROWA.
88. Western Australia Public Health Department. 1936. *Report of the Public Health Department for the years 1935 and 1936*. Perth: Department of Public Health, 8.
89. Davis to Atkinson, September 9, 1936 (Cons 1003, PHD, 1935/0732), SROWA.
90. Ibid.
91. Kidd, Rosalind. 2005. *The Way We Civilise*. St Lucia: University of Queensland Press, 113.
92. Ibid., 115.
93. Cited in ibid., 114.
94. Queensland Department of Health. 1937. *Annual Report on the Health and Medical Services of the State of Queensland for the year 1936–1937*. Brisbane: The State, 11.
95. 'National Health and Medical Research Council, 1st Session, February 1937,' *MJA*. March 6, 1937, 382.
96. Cilento, R.W. 1938. 'Leprosy in Queensland.' In Department of Health and Home Affairs, *Annual Report on the Health and Medical Services of the State of Queensland for the year 1937–1938*. Brisbane: The State, 16.
97. Ibid.
98. Ibid., 16, 12.
99. Section 51, *Health Act* 1937 (QLD).
100. Queensland Department of Health. 1939. *Annual Report on the Health and Medical Services of the State of Queensland for the year 1938–1939*. Brisbane: The State, 128.
101. Ibid., 129.
102. 'Interim Report to Sir Cilento on the Leprosy Investigation of North Queensland under the NHMRC,' 28 April 1939 (Health and Medical Services Branch, A388, Papers, ITM8887), Queensland State Archives (QSA).
103. Croll, Graham. 'Interim Report on the Investigation of Leprosy among Aborigines in North Queensland, 25 October 1939, submitted to NHMRC November 1939' (A388, ITM8887), QSA.

CHAPTER 4

The Church, the State, and Missionary Women

In March 1932, Australia's Prime Minister, Joseph Lyons, received a letter from the Provincial Superior of the Sisters of St John of God in the Kimberley, Western Australia. She asked him to support the Sisters' application for nursing work at Channel Island leprosarium in the Northern Territory. Further requests followed in the 1930s, all unsuccessful. The Sisters' persistence reflected their desire to maintain the care and evangelisation of leprosy patients from Beagle Bay Mission, who under new government policy, had been sent north. The Sisters were well-qualified, having had long missionary experience with Indigenous people in the Kimberley, and nurse training. But however attractive the terms offered, authorities were unwilling to appoint Catholic Sisters to the role at that time. This would not remain so. By the early 1940s, the three Indigenous leprosaria would be staffed by Catholic Sisters. What changed? Intersecting developments in train by the late interwar period coalesced: the changed focus of international and domestic Catholic missionaries; the increasing interest of veiled Catholic women in particular in the Indigenous missions, and shifts in the policies of Indigenous affairs bureaucracies. Another factor to emerge during World War II was the shortages of lay nurses.

C. Robson, *Missionary Women, Leprosy and Indigenous Australians, 1936–1986*, https://doi.org/10.1007/978-3-031-05796-0_4

The Australian Catholic Missionary Imperative of the Interwar Period

From about 1914, the Vatican began encouraging Catholic missionaries to evangelise Indigenous Australians with the appointment of the first apostolic delegate to Australia, Bonaventura Cerretti who claimed to have received direct instructions from the Propaganda del Fide (the central Catholic missions agency of the Vatican) regarding 'the Aborigines of the Country.' But responses by bishops were slow and required more encouragement.[1] In 1926, Pope Pius XI's encyclical, *Rerum Ecclesiae*, exhorted Catholic clergy to spread the faith to indigenous peoples worldwide. "Guiding and protecting the Lord's Flock" was not enough; they must "strive by might and main to win over and to join to Christ all who are still without the Fold." Priests were urged to establish more mission stations, develop "native clergy," and were cautioned, "Anyone who looks upon these natives as members of an inferior race or as men of low mentality makes a grievous mistake."[2]

In response, the Northern Australian mission fields saw a significant increase in male and female Catholic religious, ultimately outnumbering their Protestant counterparts. Initially, a few enthusiastic bishops and priests took up the call from Rome, their awakened sense of duty to the Indigenous race in parallel with more generalised concerns expressed concomitantly in Australia. New remote mission stations were established and seminarians' journals encouraged Australian and Irish-born priests and Brothers to join their German and French confreres who made up the majority of missionary personnel. The Pallottine Fathers opened a new seminary in Kew, Victoria in 1937 to train Australian men for the Kimberley missions, and the Indigenous missionary cause featured in magazines from the 1930s to inform the Catholic community and to elicit their financial support.[3]

The Australian Eucharistic Congresses of 1934 and 1938 were showcases of Catholic missionary achievement. Like the Vatican Missionary Exhibition on which they were modelled, they were designed to encourage vocations and funding for the missions. Catholic mission pioneers, Bishops Raible of the Kimberley and Gsell of Darwin and Father Patrick Moloney of Central Australia addressed the 1938 Congress on their individual endeavours, hoping to refute the assertion, in Moloney's words, that "nothing can be done with the Abo":

> If Dr Raible had addressed us on the Africans, Maoris or Papuans, you would not have been surprised at the success of Catholicity among any of those people, but that Australian Aborigines readily accept the Faith, and make such good Catholics, you are surprised...[4]

Moloney was known in his order, the Missionaries of the Sacred Heart (MSC), for his energy and determination for the missionary cause, which he discovered at a relatively late stage of life. When not on the missions, he was extolling their virtues to brothers and priests with speeches, retreats, and articles; chastising Catholics for their indifference; and writing to governments for mission subsidies.

This new upsurge in Catholic missionary zeal led to a marked increase in Catholic mission stations in remote Australia from the 1920s. The lion's share belonged to the MSC which, in the decade from 1929, opened missions at Port Keats, Melville Island, Alice Springs, and Tennant Creek in the Northern Territory, and Palm and Hammond Islands in northern Queensland. In northern Western Australia, in the same period, the Pallottine Fathers opened a mission at Rockhole, bringing the number of missions they operated in the Kimberley to four.[5] The trend continued into the next decade so that by 1944, seventy-four Catholic missionaries were attached to nine mission stations, compared with twenty-five Presbyterian and twenty Anglican missionaries at six and five mission stations respectively. Only the interdenominational society, the United Aborigines Mission, had more missionaries than the Catholics.[6] A high proportion of the Catholic influx were women, as Sisters were often appointed in groups of two or more, to teach, nurse, and housekeep.

While Catholic women missionaries were largely dependent for their work on the establishment of mission stations by priests, mission stations could not flourish without the participation of women. They brought domestic and teaching skills, but nursing, more particularly, was a valued female skill, and advantageous in the Indigenous mission field, where infectious diseases, infant and maternal health problems, and nutritional deficiencies prevailed. Moreover, *Rerum Ecclesiae* urged missionaries to minister to the health needs of their charges before preaching the gospel, as Christ had done: "...missionaries who preach to the heathen know only too well how much good-will and real affection is gained for the Church by those who look after the health of the natives and care for their sick..."[7] However, Catholic missionaries' capacity to heed this papal directive was constrained by a concomitant ban on their attendance at maternity cases and the practice of medicine and surgery, under separate papal decrees of 1901 and 1917, respectively.[8] These rules officially excluded Catholic missionary health carers from practising midwifery and postnatal care, placing them at a disadvantage compared with Protestant missionaries. In February 1936, the Vatican issued *Constans ac Sedula* which lifted the bans and encouraged female religious to practice maternity and paediatric nursing to bring Catholic missionaries on the same footing as other nurses.[9]

The Sisters of St John of God, the Kimberley, Western Australia

The Kimberley community of the Sisters of St John of God (SSJG) had been working with Indigenous people in the north long before the interwar Catholic mission upsurge. They would play a significant role in Australian leprosy caregiving, serving at Derby leprosarium and, through offshoot community, the Our Lady Help of Christians (OLHC), at Fantome Island. Even after another order, the Franciscan Missionaries of Mary, took over nursing on the Island, some OLHC sisters changed to that order to maintain their positions.

Nursing was always central to the SSJG apostolate. The origins can be traced back to the Bon Secours, a French female congregation founded in 1824 in Paris, whose members were principally engaged in home nursing for the wealthy. New communities were established in Ireland in 1861 but, before long, conflict arose, due partly to the reluctance of some women to care for the privileged in the midst of surrounding poverty. Several Sisters, led by Sister Brigid Clancy, left the order and formed a new congregation under Bishop Thomas Furlong who had sought a nursing community to care for the sick poor in his diocese of Ferns, Co. Wexford. Furlong named the congregation after the sixteenth-century John Ciudad of Portugal (aka St John of God), whose life was to serve as a model for the Irish Sisters. Ciudad has been depicted as self-sacrificing and egalitarian, devoted to the sick poor, and forward thinking in his incorporation of hygiene practices in his hospital. The St John of God Sisters nursed in homes, workhouses, and infirmaries, later adding school-teaching to their activities, as included in their first constitution.[10]

The Sisters' arrival in Australia followed a request by Bishop Matthew Gibney of Perth for nurses to attend a typhoid fever outbreak on the Coolgardie and Kalgoorlie goldfields of Western Australia in 1895. This role brought the Sisters to primitive conditions, nursing in tents with the heat and dust, and the threat of contracting this highly infectious disease. At Kalgoorlie, the SSJG established their first Australian base and a hospital that became an early nurse training school for both religious and lay nurses in 1909. The first novitiate, the motherhouse, and another hospital were opened at Subiaco, Perth, in 1898.[11]

In 1907, the SSJG began work with Indigenous Australians when some Sisters joined the Pallottine Fathers' Beagle Bay Mission to provide education and maternal care for the young residents. The Wexford motherhouse and the Subiaco community opposed this move, and disassociated the Sisters from their congregation, leaving the latter dependent on the priests for their upkeep.[12] Fresh recruits were drawn from Ireland for the mission including two of the Greene family of County Clare, Emilia (Sister Bernadine), and Susan (Sister Brigid). In subsequent years, three more siblings followed: Anne, Catherine, and Margaret (Sisters Gertrude, Matthew and Gabriel, respectively), and also Margaret Carmody. Historian Pat Jacobs has remarked on the "cultural transfer" with the introduction of Irish Catholicism, music and singing to the children by the Sisters.[13] German priests and brothers brought another cultural influence. Beagle Bay, therefore, was insulated from mainstream Anglo-Australian society and culture in the early part of the twentieth century. Close relationships developed between the Sisters and the mission people, many of whom adopted the Catholic faith and continued to work for and support the mission as adults.[14] Several married and passed their children to the care of the Sisters who acted as surrogate mothers, nursed and taught while their young charges worked in the farm, laundry and kitchen.[15] Thus mutual interdependence and close relations developed between whole families and the Sisters.

In 1908, Mother Antonio, seeking independence for her Sisters from the Pallottine Fathers, headed north up the Dampierland coast to Broome. With just one other Sister and without support from her Church, she opened another convent which, according to scholar and SSJG Sister, Pat Rhatigan, "formed the base from which they could independently shape their apostolate to the Aboriginal people as they saw fit."[16] The women initiated a programme of charitable works primarily in the fields of education and nursing. At this time, Broome had a thriving pearling industry and was home to diverse races, including Japanese, Filipinos, Chinese, and Irish. Some, especially the Filipinos, provided material assistance to the Sisters and became part of the religious community that grew around their activities.[17] The Sisters nursed typhoid victims in the Japanese hospital and taught the children of settlers of different nationalities. Indigenous people, however, were largely excluded from this multiracial society; legislation prohibited their entry to the Broome township except for employment.[18] One Sister remembered it was not until at least World War I that "the natives filtered into Broome…and our school [St Mary's] gradually became a coloured school."[19]

The Australian foundations of the SSJG continued to recruit postulants from Ireland throughout the twentieth century but were always short of numbers required as mission stations increased. In 1912, the Kimberley Sisters, worried about their ageing community and its ability to continue the challenging work, initiated a recruitment drive in the south-eastern states. Mother Bernadine Greene secured eight young "strong, happy, efficient Australians."[20] Hope was invested in these women, all from cities and country towns of New South Wales and Victoria, to cope with the inherent difficulties of missionary work in the remote north-west.[21] Greene further noted with delight that several women were trained in fields prized in the Sisters' apostolate: Eileen Murnane (Sister Ignatius), a trained teacher; nineteen-year-old Kathleen Daly (Sister Alphonsus), a musician; a trained nurse and some "fairly good singers."[22]

From about the mid-1920s, the internal organisation of the Kimberley SSJG underwent destabilisation, and its Indigenous mission work came under threat. To centralise international SSJG administration, the Subiaco province was formally amalgamated with the motherhouse in Wexford. The Kimberley Sisters were invited to join Subiaco on condition they relinquish the Indigenous missions. Mission pioneers, Antonio O'Brien and Bernadine Greene had both died in 1923. Magdalen Cashen, then in charge of three small foundations in the north-west, was the major figure in ensuing negotiations. She and her cohort were as determined as the previous generation to retain mission work, and they refused Subiaco's demands. Kimberley bishop, Ernest Coppo, suggested the stranded community be saved through incorporation into the Salesian Daughters of Mary Help of Christians, an Italian congregation, and thereby retain their missionary work. Sydney Archbishop Michael Kelly would provide a Sydney novitiate and base for the Sisters in return for their taking up domestic duties at St Columba's seminary in Sydney's Blue Mountains. Sister Ignatius led a group of Sisters to Sydney in 1926 and began work. The merger with the Salesians did not go ahead but the Sisters formed a new congregation in 1931, the OLHC, under Kelly's episcopal control, with his promise of mission work when available. Several SSJG Sisters left the Kimberley to join the OLHC including, from the 1912 cohort, Cashen and Murnane, who was made Superior. Despite missionary ambitions, they remained in seminary work either indefinitely or for many years.[23]

In 1929, Wexford agreed to amalgamate the much-depleted Kimberley community with the SSJG congregation as a separate province. The Sisters could continue missionary work but were forbidden to perform maternal nursing and advised to employ lay midwives instead.[24] The reiteration of this canonical restriction suggests that it was probably flouted by the Sisters at times. Far from medical services and faced with life-threatening deliveries, their transgressions were not hard to understand.

The Sisters of St John of God and the Leprosy Apostolate

Shortly before Channel Island leprosarium opened in 1931, the Kimberley SSJG applied for the nursing roles. Sister Gertrude wrote to Albert Green, the Federal Member for Kalgoorlie, whom she knew from her nursing days in the goldfields. She stressed the Sisters' nursing experience and their relationships with the leprosy patients at Beagle Bay Mission. The Sisters would be sorry to lose them to Channel Island, a secular institution, as many were under Catholic instruction.[25]

Green supported her application, describing the Sisters glowingly to the Minister for Home Affairs, as "…a very fine body of women who are used to the tropical climate."[26] Sister Gertrude had also written twice to Prime Minister James Scullin, perhaps as one devout Irish Catholic to another. But the requests were in vain. The lay curator and matron were already undergoing training and the leprosarium would open the following month[27] (Fig. 4.1).

The following year, Father William Henschke MSC, who, as Darwin parish priest, visited Channel Island regularly, told the Kimberley Sisters that the lay staff was "tired of the place," and the Sisters' Superior wrote to the Prime Minister, then Joseph Lyons:

> We are writing to say that we will be very pleased to take charge of it and could send three sisters one of whom at least would be a trained nurse. We are a nursing order and have sisters with the ASNA certificate. We have

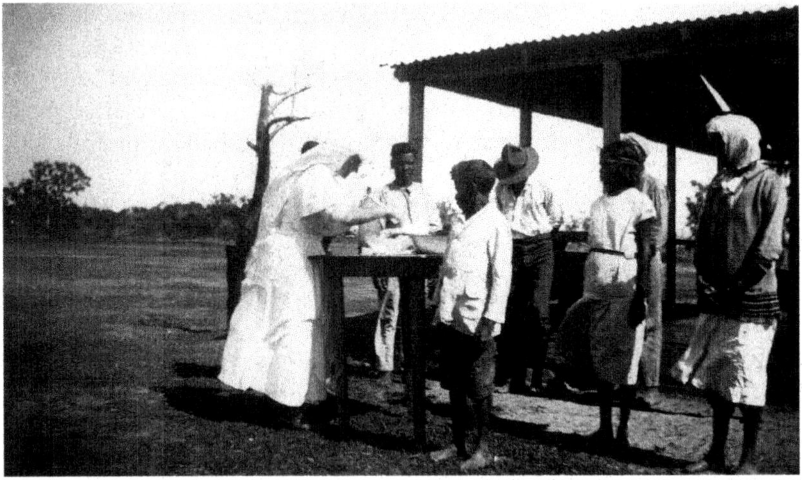

Fig. 4.1 Sr Brigid Greene and leprosy patients at Beagle Bay Mission temporary lazaret, 1930–1936 (SSJG Heritage Centre Broome)

> been engaged on the Black Missions for the past 25 years so that we have a good experience in nursing Blacks. I understand that food and medicine are supplied by the Government. We would need a yearly sum for clothing and incidentals. We could not pay the way of the sisters or supply furniture as we have no funds. We would take it as a great favour if you would help us in this matter.[28]

The Sisters' terms were generous, and they brought considerable experience. Lyons, yet another Catholic, might have been sympathetic to their request. But the government declined their offer again, explaining that no vacancy had arisen.[29] Over the next two years, the Sisters, with Henschke as advocate, continued to press their case, but to no avail. Although the ultimate decision on staffing lay with the federal government, its officers looked to the advice of Cecil Cook, the Chief Medical Officer of the Northern Territory.[30] In late 1933, when the current staff resigned, the Sisters' applications received serious consideration. Cook was, however,

> wholeheartedly opposed to this method of staffing ...Where an Institution is controlled by one authority and staffed by an outside organisation over which that authority has no control... Change of personnel in the Roman

> Catholic Presbytery may easily be followed by conflict of policy between the Chief Medical Officer and the co-religionists of the Orders staffing the Leprosarium. It is not sufficient to meet this possibility with the assurance that in the event of the Chief Medical Officer being dissatisfied, the staffing arrangement will cease as I am of opinion that democratic government would prefer to solve the problem by dismissing its Chief Medical Officer.[31]

As Suzanne Saunders has argued, this letter suggests Cook's central objection was the potential for his own "loss of control."[32] Leprosarium policy had been his from its inception, and he evidently believed government employees, who presumably had no higher authorities to serve, were the only means to have his ideas carried out.

Nevertheless, the negotiations continued. The Northern Territory Administrator and the Secretary of the Department of the Interior supported the Sisters, one having been nursed by the SSJG, and the other convinced of "their sincerity and devotion to duty."[33] With Henschke, they produced a proposal for federal Cabinet in May 1934. Cook's main objection was addressed with an assurance from the Sisters to "carry out implicitly and without question the directions of the Chief Medical Officer."[34] The final plan was to engage four Sisters with nursing experience, including one with qualifications, and a Brother as superintendent, as authorities considered a male staff member essential in a mixed institution. Remuneration of the religious staff was about £200 per annum cheaper than for the lay staff but an initial additional £3200 was needed to construct accommodation for the extra personnel.[35]

Two weeks later, Henschke was told that the Sisters would not be appointed as the construction costs were too expensive, and anyway, not worth the trouble: since the leprosarium was insufficient to accommodate escalating Western Australian cases, a larger replacement institution was under consideration.[36] He doubted the reason given, since the Sisters would have tolerated the existing accommodation.[37] Possibly Cook's views prevailed, but giving financial reasons was more diplomatic.

Cook's objections to the Sisters' involvement were also likely related to his general disapproval of missionaries as health carers. He was critical of carelessness and incompetence in missions and complained that residents with infectious diseases were not properly quarantined, thereby increasing the spread of leprosy.[38] Cook was adamant that formal nursing qualifications in Indigenous health settings were essential. In the leprosarium, qualified nurses were required, especially to deal with obstetric emergencies as medical help was too far away, and women with leprosy often experienced dangerous pregnancies and childbirth.[39] Catholic Sisters, being constrained from performing these duties under canonical prohibitions, were unsuitable. Cook makes no mention of this issue in 1934, but it was raised as a reason for his objections by Sister Gertrude in a letter to him over a decade later.[40]

The SSJG needed only to wait two more years before the opportunity for leprosy nursing re-emerged, with the opening of the Derby leprosarium in the Kimberley. Several factors worked in their favour this time. First, in 1936, the Vatican lifted the bans on attending childbirth and postnatal care by Catholic religious. Sister Gertrude immediately undertook further training and acquired certificates in midwifery, infant welfare and mothercraft.[41] Second, in March 1937, after a few months as leprosarium staff, the Luyers left, following strained relations with the Derby Medical Officer, Albert Davis. Shortly after, Sisters Gertrude and Brigid Greene arrived to temporarily take on the nursing.[42]

After three months, their Provincial Superior, Mother Margaret Carmody negotiated a permanent arrangement with Under-Secretary, Frederick Huelin:

> I gathered that your Order was agreeable to provide permanently the nursing staff at the leprosarium. You will, from time to time, exchange one nurse for another, but you will be willing to maintain the necessary nursing services for the patients. I would like to say that the Hon. Minister and the Department thankfully accept this offer. We know what it means to you, and it is really difficult to express our appreciation of the self-sacrificing service on the part of your Sisterhood that this offer involves.[43]

The main benefit for the government was the stabilisation of leprosarium nursing services, as Huelin explained in a handwritten note to the Treasurer: "We have no worry about securing staff which would be very difficult - no annual leave, no relievers, no steamer fares!!"[44] But the government did have to pay for their services. For two nurses, the remuneration was £390 per annum plus food and lodgings, an amount exceeding wages for many Australian registered nurses at the time, but below those for the Channel Island matron. In line with the Sisters' vow of poverty, the payment was remitted not to them personally but to their community.[45] For the government, the payment for the Sisters' labour ensured control over their performance: "our position is safeguarded by the fact that the nurses are paid servants of this department."[46]

Securing the Derby leprosarium nursing work was something of a victory for both the SSJG community and Australian Catholic missionaries generally. It crowned a decade of failed attempts by missionaries of various denominations to be permitted an official part in leprosy care. Apart from the leprosarium in New Guinea, Derby leprosarium was the first instance in which an Australian government had placed Christian religious on its payroll. Certainly, options were limited, other than to appoint the few trained nursing Sisters in the north-west willing to do the work. But the preparedness of the SSJG should not be discounted as an equal factor in effecting this arrangement. Being available and suitably qualified as leprosy struck the heartland of their missionary activity reflected the Church's growing interest in the Indigenous missions and its mobilisation of the necessary personnel. In addition, the Kimberley Sisters' own persistent ambitions to acquire and maintain the Indigenous apostolate was an important factor.

The Our Lady Help of Christians and Fantome Island

The leprosarium for 'coloured' people in the Palm Island group in northern Queensland presented a second opportunity for Archbishop Kelly to honour his promise of Indigenous missionary work to the sisters who had left SSJG to form the OLHC. The first had been in 1934, when Sisters Ignatius Murnane and Magdalen Cashen joined the Palm Island Catholic mission to teach and evangelise the community. Initially, the Daughters of Our Lady of the Sacred Heart (DOLSH) had been strong contenders for this mission as it was founded and continued to be run by their filial congregation, the MSC. Kelly, however, over-rode such considerations to honour his pledge. The OLHC, having then a base on Palm Island, were the obvious choice when the leprosarium was opened six years later.

The issue of nursing staff at Fantome Island was raised early in the planning stage. The Queensland Protector of Aboriginals, J.W. Bleakley, suggested the matron-curator model as at Channel Island but the Director-General of Health, Raphael Cilento, believed qualified lay nurses would be difficult to obtain, especially with wartime shortages.[47] He suggested Catholic Sister nurses, and, after permission from

E.M. Hanlon, the Minister for Home and Health Affairs, approached the Catholic bishop of Townsville, Hugh Ryan, in September 1939. Ryan contacted Mother Ignatius, who provided four nurses for the leprosarium.[48]

The negotiations for engaging the Sisters went smoothly as both Hanlon and Bleakley, a strong advocate of Christian missions, were supportive. In a government propaganda publication of the late 1930s, Hanlon "and his lieutenant, the Chief Protector" were said to be improving the material welfare and health of Queensland Indigenous people to save them from extinction by entrusting the missions with their care. "…all serve the Government nobly in maintaining a humane and fatherly care over these remnants of our black race."[49] The pamphlet referred to the rising prevalence of leprosy in Queensland Indigenous people and the danger of "allowing them to mingle indiscriminately with whites."[50] So taken was Hanlon with the Catholic Sisters that within two months of their arrival at Fantome Island, he suggested they be granted full control of both the leprosarium and the lock hospital.[51]

Closer analysis of Cilento's reasons for requesting the services of the Sisters reveals that their nursing qualifications were not the only deciding factor. Cilento, on visiting leprosy facilities at Makogai in Fiji and Anelaua in New Guinea, admired the professionalism and dedication of the Catholic Sisters on staff, and assumed such qualities were common to Catholic Sister nurses.[52] He didn't seem to share Cook's concern about their potential to disregard medical authority. But, unlike Cilento, Cook's contact with Catholic religious had been in the missions whereas Cilento's was almost certainly confined to tropical health institutions.[53] Cilento was enthusiastic about engaging religious Sisters and wrote approvingly to Bishop Ryan of leprosy research at Makogai: "Several of the Sisters at Makogai have become very expert in this direction and one or two, I believe, have even published their observations on the matter."[54] The Sisters were envisaged as researchers as well as nurses; collaborators in Cilento's vision.

Cilento also valued the Sisters for their presumed chasteness. His strong disapproval of a lay nurse's flirtatious behaviour with the Indigenous men on Palm Island has been discussed by historian Hilary Carey. The contrast between the nurse's sexual expressiveness and the modest unobtrusiveness of the Makogai Sisters must have been striking to Cilento. The religious vow of celibacy allowed the work to be fulfilled, undistracted, as Carey put it, "without exciting the anxiety about sexual contact habitually invoked by the casual association of white women and black men in a tropical environment."[55] Apart from any moral abhorrence Cilento may have had for interracial sexual relations, sex between carer and patient was seen as unprofessional and conducive to the spread of disease, considering the theoretical link between sexual intimacy and leprosy proposed by Cook.

Finally, the financial savings, if not Cilento's primary reason, were appealing to his departmental superiors. Each Sister was paid £50 per annum, increasing by £1 for every patient over the number of fifty. In March 1940, four Sisters had charge of seventy-five patients, giving an annual payment of just £75 per Sister.[56] It was about half the salary offered for the nursing position at the island's lock hospital being advertised at the same time, appended with a postscript that the appointee "will not be required for duty at the recently established leprosarium."[57]

Unlike the Irish, mostly middle-aged Sisters who staffed Derby, the four OLHC Sisters who commenced nursing at Fantome Island in 1940 were Australian-born and three out of four were young. Sisters Catherine, Bernadette and Agnes were aged between 21 and 23, while the Superior, Mother Peter, was 42. They had no previous connection with the patients or their communities, nor could the younger ones have had much, if any, missionary experience. The missionary impulse, however, was evident in the "special purposes" of the OLHC constitution, the "conversion and education of pagans and especially of Australian Aboriginals" as well as their community's ethos, carried over from the former SSJG Sisters who became their superiors and novice mistresses.[58] To a greater extent than for Derby, the Fantome Island leprosarium work was part of a wider missionary initiative by the Church, being brokered and supported by the Sydney and Townsville dioceses.

The Daughters of Our Lady of the Sacred Heart and the Channel Island Leprosarium

In February 1942, after the bombing of Darwin by the Japanese, Channel Island leprosarium was evacuated under advice from senior medical officer, Bruce Kirkland. With no red crosses on the rooves of its buildings, the leprosarium resembled a military base from the air, opening it to attack. The patients had been excluded from the general evacuation of the Darwin area the previous December, as nobody wanted to transport potentially infectious people.[59] Matron Elsie Jones had fallen seriously ill and she and her husband Jack had left.[60] The seventy or so patients were given camping equipment and two months of rations, before crossing the mud flats to the mainland and disappearing into the bush.

In March, the Northern Territory was placed under military command, and some months later, fearing the troops could be infected with leprosy, the Army located most of the patients and returned them to Channel Island.[61] By January 1943, Kirkland had resumed their medical treatment, but had no staff to care for the patients. A letter from the Deputy Director of Medical Services of the Northern Territory Armed Forces (DDMS) to his superior explains the difficulties:

> The Roman Catholic bishop of Northern Territory has been approached and is willing to provide two trained nuns to live on the island and help with the treatment. The GOC [General Commanding Officer] is willing that women be allowed to live on the island but he will not guarantee their evacuation in the event of an attack, but he will do his best to have them brought off in time to avoid capture by the enemy. The GOC has given DDMS permission to write this letter but insists that the DGMS [Director General of Medical Services] be made conversant with the fact that it may raise a denominational fracas.[62]

J.H.L. Cumpston, the Commonwealth Director-General of Health, favoured the proposal. He doubted sectarian friction would occur or that the Japanese would land on the island as they were reputed to be frightened of leprosy.[63]

In April, two DOLSH Sisters, Gabriella Formarick and Campion Bryant arrived from Sydney to begin nursing on the island. Both were experienced and qualified nursing Sisters, Formarick having worked at Bathurst Island Mission and Bryant at Nauru from where she had been recently evacuated.[64] While the war continued, they were not remunerated for their services, but were given a "uniform allowance" of ten shillings each per week.[65]

When the Army had first suggested Sisters for the leprosarium, Bishop Gsell and Fr Henschke had immediately recommended the DOLSH, who had worked in missions and schools in the region prior to the outbreak of war, and were the filial congregation of their own order, the MSC. Henschke was particularly eager to see Catholic sisters at Channel Island after his failed attempts with the SSJG a decade earlier. The fact that his sibling, Mother Concepta, was Superior of the Australian Province of DOLSH, would not have hurt his chances of success this time.

The DOLSH was founded in Issoudun, France in 1874 by Jules Chevalier. Their original apostolate centred on the education of girls and "other works of charity" as well as spiritual contemplation. In 1883, after the Pope had directed the MSCs to New Guinea for their first overseas missionary work, the DOLSH amended their constitution to include work in the "Foreign Missions," with the intention of joining the priests.[66] Such ventures were normally voluntary for Catholic Sisters, despite the vow of obedience they took. However, the congregation inserted a fourth optional vow in their updated constitution, that, if sworn, obliged Sisters to "go to the foreign missions at the command of the Superiors of the Congregation and that not withstanding [sic] the perils, sacrifices of all kinds and even death itself which may await them"[67] (Fig. 4.2).

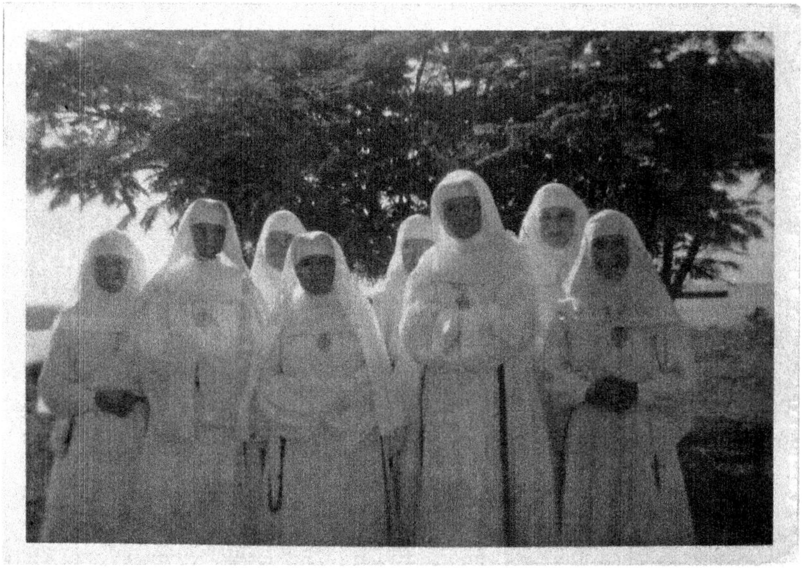

Fig. 4.2 Sisters at Channel Island Leprosarium 1955. Back row: Virginia Harper, Eucharia Pearce, Anthony Menhinnitt, Daniel Kennedy. Front row: Benedicta Carroll, Florine Gimson, Concepta Henschke (Provincial Superior), Columbanus Baker (DOLSH Archives, Kensington, NSW)

The DOLSH Sisters left France in 1885 to work in the Pacific islands with the MSCs, stopping in Sydney *en route*. There they were waylaid by the parish priest and asked to stay and open schools in the local suburbs of Botany and Randwick. Some Sisters also established a school on Thursday Island, the intended base for the MSC Melanesian mission operations. In the 1880s and 1890s, Sisters finally joined these missions and went on to open schools and novitiates throughout Australia.[68]

Increasingly, Australian women entered the congregation, eventually replacing their French predecessors, and a large convent was built at Kensington beside the MSC Sydney provincial headquarters. The Sisters did not necessarily regard their focus on schools as divergent to their central missionary goals, for schools potentially trained future missionaries. Until 1912, the only missionary work undertaken by the Sisters was in the Pacific region. In 1908, after the MSCs became established in the Northern Territory, the DOLSH began teaching the Catholic (non-Indigenous) population of Darwin at Gsell's request. Four years later, they joined him on Bathurst Island to undertake the evangelisation of the Tiwi people.[69]

The DOLSH congregation's traditional links with missionary work were articulated in its 1928 constitution:

> The first work of zeal for which the Institute was at its beginning designed and destined is that of the Missions among the Infidels. ...the Sisters will assist the Missionaries in all their works of Charity and Apostleship as far as their sex, their profession and Constitutions permit; this is their principal work.[70]

While this direction implies that the Sisters were to take a supplementary role to the male missionary, the Constitutions also specify "instructing the natives," confirming the Sisters' evangelising role at mission stations,

> ...to be called to make God known to these savages in spite of the degree of ignorance they are in is no ordinary grace, and to raise them from the base ideas in which they are plunged to Christian ideals is no small thing.[71]

The Sisters became part of the expanding network of MSC Northern Territory missions: Alice Springs, Port Keats, Melville Island, Daly River. Nursing did not become a major apostolate in Australia for the DOLSH until after the papal ban on obstetric nursing was lifted in 1936. Two years later, Sister Gabriella Formarick became Bathurst Island's first trained nurse which afforded her appropriate experience when she began at Channel Island seven years later.[72]

Individual Vocations

What of the individual Sisters' personal aspirations? Can they be fairly represented in the rules and actions of their congregation? And how persuasive were the Church's recruitment strategies of the post World War I era? Oral and written testimonies provided by former leprosarium Sisters indicate that, for many, missionary endeavour among non-Christian peoples had long been a personal ambition and had prompted their decision to join a religious community. Some particularly wanted to work with Indigenous Australians; for others, the distinction wasn't made. Sister Benedicta Carroll OLSH, who began nursing at Channel Island in 1947 stated, "I chose this Order because of the missions."[73] Sister Marion, her successor, "had a vague feeling about missions" and thought she'd "rather like to work with the Aboriginals."[74] Sister Helene Cresp was first a lay nurse in the Northern Territory and joined the DOLSH in 1943 to become a missionary.[75] Derby leprosarium Sisters had similar ambitions although Sisters Alphonsus Daly, Ignatius Murnane (1912 entrants), and Angela Moroney (1931) joined the SSJG to work in the far northwest. Sister Alphonsus remembers her enthusiasm for evangelisation as a nineteen-year-old postulant: "We were in for a purpose; to convert the world."[76] Hilary Carey's research into the motivations of the OLHC Sisters of Fantome and Palm Islands yielded similar results. One Sister "always had missions in mind," another "always wanted to teach Aborigines," and a third, attracted by stories of Father Damien, decided at age 14 to become a missionary.[77]

The motivations of Catholic Sisters were the same, regardless of when they entered their religious community. Sister Benedicta and Sister "Jeanne," a later DOLSH entrant, considered themselves lucky to be sent to the remote missions.[78] Indeed, the 1928 Constitutions depict works undertaken "at home" as ancillary to missionary work—reserved for those too young or frail, or in need of a break from the demands of the missions.[79] Yet only a little more than one third of these women pursued a missionary vocation, as most took up teaching positions in local parishes.[80] While probably not all DOLSH entrants aimed for a missionary vocation, those who did so did not all have their ambitions satisfied, either because they were deemed unsuitable physically or mentally, or because the concurrent demands of the parish exceeded those of the mission fields (Fig. 4.3).

Often the perception of "missions" was drawn from the experiences of those who had preceded them into the mission fields: inspirational talks; items in missionary society magazines; and hagiographies of saints or respected missionaries, such as St Francis of Assisi and Father Damien.[81] Sister Marion ascribed her decision to become a religious to a lecture by a missionary priest in the Northern Territory.

> I was very impressed at the talk he gave and the way he spoke about the Sisters who worked with him, and how helpful they were, and what wonderful work they did, and I thought to myself, I'd never really heard a priest speak like that about any Sisters.[82]

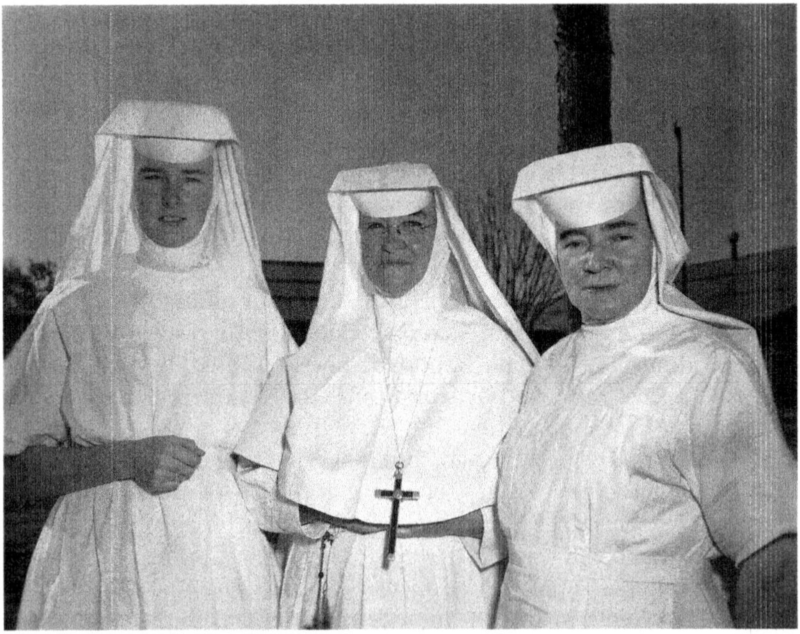

Fig. 4.3 Derby Leprosarium Sisters n.d. Left to right: Mechtilde Crosby, Alphonsus Daly, Angela Moroney (SSJG Heritage Centre Broome)

So, although she had heard of admirable male missionaries, it was only during this talk that she discovered an avenue for herself, as a woman, to pursue a valuable missionary career. The conceptualisation of such a role depended on the successful construction of an image of a population in need. The human suffering conveyed in missionary propaganda and recruiting drives and the offer of a chance to remedy it was evidently a powerful inducement to female aspirants.

Tapping into female maternal urges was one means of attracting women to the mission cause. Promotional material for the remote north missions featured emotive images of Indigenous infants or young children. Sometimes a religious Sister was shown holding a child with the mother absent from the image, as if, often deceptively, she did not exist. Such images and the accompanying literature targeted single Australian women, subtly, promising a maternal role without the obligations of marriage. This kind of publicity persuaded leprosarium nurse, Sister Angela Moroney SJG and missionary Sister, Mary Molloy OLHC to join their orders in 1927 and 1945 respectively.[83] Although from an early age Moroney had "wanted to become a missionary and look after black babies," her defining moment came when she saw, in a Catholic newspaper, "a pathetic picture of three black babies with very skinny limbs" beside a request for mission recruits from the Kimberley SSJG.[84]

Like the 'orphans' in mission magazines, leprosy-affected people were also depicted as needing to be rescued by Catholic Sisters. Classic portrayals of the outcast, unsightly 'leper' were used to amplify the opportunities for the missionary cause. Yet, this depiction masked the reality in which Indigenous patients were not shunned by their communities but had been removed under public health regulations. The leprosarium Sisters and priests were likened to the idolised Damien of Molokai and the leprosarium apostolate figured as a dramatic example of pious and rewarding missionary vocations among "the most afflicted and abandoned of our Aboriginal population."[85]

To respond to these recruiting overtures was a courageous, but not entirely uncharacteristic step for single women in the first half of the twentieth century. Many headed off to pursue adventurous yet dutiful, if sometimes short-lived, careers in the armed forces, the Red Cross, and Protestant Christian mission ventures.[86] They exchanged a more conventional life of family and domesticity for one of risk and unpredictability. With fewer men present, they relied on their own skills, experience, and sometimes other women's support.

Whether from the Australian rural towns and cities or from overseas, women entering the remote missions faced radical changes to their lives. Snakes, mosquitoes, fevers, floods, cyclones, extreme heat, and water and food shortages would be the order of the day. Yet, they could still experience freedoms denied to most Catholic Sisters of this period, as described here by Naomi Turner:

> Until and beyond the 1960s the religious sister was seen as belonging either to the school or to the hospital. She wore black and brown medieval clothing and veil, and rarely moved out of her convent; and when she did, it was in company with another sister. Her life was rigidly organised into a daily pattern of work and prayer.[87]

Nursing qualifications became key assets for religious Sisters and their communities to access mission fields, and, as we have seen, leprosy work. For that reason, many Sisters were chosen by their Provincials to train as nurses after they had joined the order with no particular apostolate in mind, except perhaps the 'missions.' They were obliged to practice nursing to the utmost of their ability, as work performed in the service of God. For women with professional nursing qualifications prior to entering the convent, on the taking of religious vows, the practice of nursing became newly framed as an expression of pious devotion. Nursing by the Sisters brought them close to their patients and could potentially engender interest in their religious faith. As DOLSH congregational historian, Sister Venard, explained, "To win these people for Christ, she first of all concerns herself with their physical ills, draws them to Him by her loving and efficient solicitude."[88] In the leprosarium, this dependence could become stronger where illness led the nurse into close and continual proximity to her patient (Fig. 4.4).

Notes

1. Livingston, K.T. 1979. 'Voices in the Wilderness: Apologists for the Aborigines in the Past.' *Australasian Catholic Record* 56 (2), 188.
2. Pope Pius XI. 1926. Rerum Ecclesiae, *The Vatican*, http://www.vatican.va/holy_father/pius_xi/encyclicals/documents/hf_p-xi_enc_28021926_rerum-ecclesiae_en.html (accessed 13 January 2010), Parts 26, 27, 29.

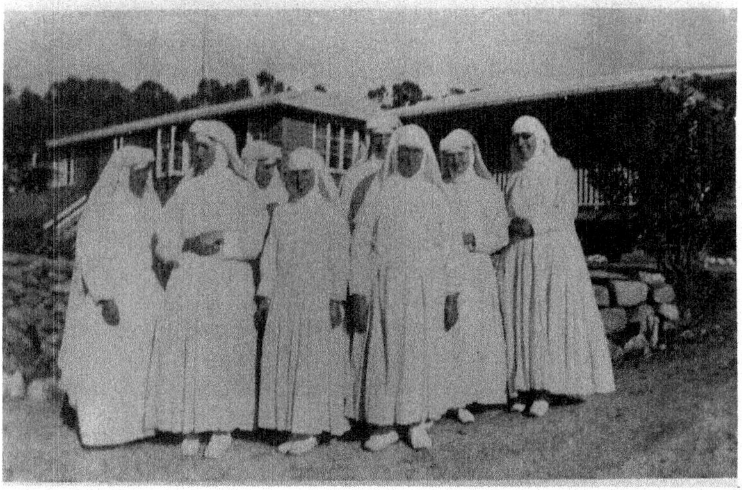

Fig. 4.4 Franciscan Missionaries of Mary Sisters at Fantome Island c. 1945 (James Cook University Library Special Collections)

3. Girola, Stefano. 2007. Rhetoric and Action: The Policies and Attitudes of the Catholic Church with Regard to Australia's Indigenous Peoples 1885–1967. Ph. D. diss., University of Queensland, 2007, 112, 125–126, 134–135; Livingston, 'Voices in the Wilderness,' 188–189.
4. Cited in Dasey, M. Edward, ed. 1944. *The Story of the Regional Missionary and the Eucharistic Congress, Newcastle, NSW, Australia, 16th–20th February 1938*. Newcastle: Specialty Publications & Sales Promotions Co. Ltd., 276–277.
5. Zucker, Margaret. 2005. *From Patrons to Partners and the Separated Children of the Kimberley: A History of the Catholic Church in the Kimberley, Western Australia*, second edition. Fremantle: University of Notre Dame Press, 84.
6. Elkin, A.P. 1944. *Citizenship for the Aborigines: A National Aboriginal Policy*, first edition. Sydney: Australasian Publishing Company Pty Ltd, 104.
7. Pius XI, Rerum Ecclesiae, part 30.
8. Hogan, Edmund. 1992. *The Irish Missionary Movement: A Historical Survey 1830-1980*. Dublin: Gill and Macmillan, 106.

9. MacGinley, M.R. 2002. *A Dynamic of Hope: Institutes of Women Religious in Australia*. Darlinghurst: Crossing Press, 286; Hogan, *The Irish Missionary Movement*, 107, 109.
10. Scally, John. 1995. *To Speed on Angels' Wings: The Story of the Sisters of St John of God*. Dublin: The Columba Press, 39–45; Rhatigan, Sister Patricia M. 2006. Holy Child Orphanage for Aboriginal Girls in Broome 1939–1962. Ph D diss., University of Notre Dame, 47.
11. Ibid., 64–66; MacGinley, *A Dynamic of Hope*, 268.
12. Scally, *To Speed on Angels' Wings*, 68, 71, 108–109.
13. Jacobs, Pat. 2001. 'Exiles in the Wilderness: The Pioneer Irish Nuns of St John of God, Beagle Bay and Broome, Western Australia: 1907-1940s.' *The Australian Journal of Irish Studies* 1, 111.
14. Nailon, Brigita. 2001. *Nothing is Wasted in the Household of God: Vincent Pallotti's Vision in Australia 1901–2001*. Richmond: Spectrum Publications, 39–40; Jacobs, 'Exiles in the Wilderness,' 110–111.
15. Choo, Christine. 2001. *Mission Girls: Aboriginal Women on Catholic Missions in the Kimberley, Western Australia, 1900–1950*. Crawley: University of Western Australia Press, 62, 156, 160–161; Lockyer, Betty. 2009. *Last Truck Out*. Broome: Magabala Books, 50–51, 59–61.
16. Rhatigan, 'Holy Child Orphanage,' 57.
17. Jacobs, 'Exiles in the Wilderness,' 12.
18. Choo, *Mission Girls*, 116.
19. Murnane, Sister Mary Ignatius. c. 1973. 'My Life as a Sister of St John of God' [S.l: s.n.]. State Library of Western Australia. 10.
20. Greene, Mother Bernadine to Bishop Torres quoted in Jacobs, Pat. 2004. 'Free Women on a Savage Frontier: St John of God Sisters on the Kimberley Pearling Coast of Western Australia.' *The Australian Journal of Irish Studies* 4, 264.
21. Murnane, Sister Mary Ignatius. n.d. 'A Chaplet of Dolours.' (Papers of Joyce Caroline Dunphy, 6140A/45, MN2305), Battye Library, Western Australia.
22. Jacobs, 'Free Women on a Savage Frontier,' 264; Murnane, 'A Chaplet of Dolours.'
23. MacGinley, M.R. 2010. *An Eloquent Witness: The Sisters of Our Lady Help of Christians*. Strathfield: St Pauls Publications, 34, 36–37, 40–45, 54.
24. Ibid., 69; Rhatigan, 'Holy Child Orphanage,' 65.
25. Greene, Sister Gertrude to the Member for Kalgoorlie, Albert E. Green, July 3, 1931 (A659, 1945/1/2887), National Archives of Australia (NAA).
26. Green, A.E. to Minister for Home Affairs, Arthur Blakeley, July 10, 1931 (A659, 1945/1/2887), NAA.
27. Blakeley to Green, July 11, 1931 (A659, 1945/1/2887), NAA.

28. McCaffery, Sister Joseph to Prime Minister Joseph Lyons, March 18, 1932 (CP103/19, 84), NAA (NASNA stands for Australasian Trained Nurses Association).
29. Minister for the Interior to Prime Minister, April 15, 1932 (CP103/19, 84), NAA.
30. Saunders, Suzanne, 1989. *'A Suitable Island Site': Leprosy in the Northern Territory and the Channel Island Leprosarium 1880–1955*. Darwin: Historical Society of the Northern Territory, 32.
31. Cook, Cecil to Northern Territory Administrator, 1934 (A659, 1945/1/2887), NAA.
32. Saunders, '*A Suitable Island Site*,' 32.
33. Weddell to Brown, March 6, 1934; Brown to Weddell, March 14, 1934. Both in (A659, 1945/1/2887), NAA.
34. Ibid.
35. Carrodus to Brown, May 1, 1934 (A659, 1945/1/2887), NAA.
36. Ibid.
37. Henschke, Fr William to Brown, July 2, 1934 (A659, 1945/1/2887), NAA.
38. Kettle, Ellen, 1991. *Health Services in the Northern Territory: A History 1824–1970*, volume one. Darwin: North Australia Research Unit, 111.
39. Duncan, M.E. 1993. 'An Historical and Clinical Review of the Interaction of Leprosy and Pregnancy: A Cycle to be Broken.' *Social Science and Medicine* 37 (4), 457.
40. Sister Gertrude to Cook, April 10, 1949 (Public Health Department (PHD), 1946/0875, Cons 1003). State Records Office Western Australia (SROWA).
41. Certificate in Child Welfare and Mothercraft for Sister Gertrude Greene (2.74B), Sisters of St John of God Archives, Broome, Western Australia (SSJGB).
42. Davis, Albert to Atkinson, Everitt, May 13, 1937 (PHD, 1935/0251, Cons 1003), SROWA; *Beagle Bay Chronicle*, February 6, 1937 (2.69U), SSJGB.
43. Huelin, Frederick to Carmody, Mother Margaret (Mother Provincial SSJG Kimberley), July 22, 1937 (PHD, 1935/0251, Cons 1003), SROWA.
44. Huelin to Under Treasurer, January 20, 1938 (PHD, 1935/0251, Cons 1003), SROWA.
45. Mother Margaret to Huelin, 9 August 1937 (PHD 1935–0251, Cons 1003), SROWA.
46. Memo of discussion. 20 July 1937 (PHD, 1935/0251, Cons 1003), SROWA.
47. Bleakley, J.W., 'Memorandum,' April 5, 1939 (Item ID 717182), Queensland State Archives (QSA); Strachan, Glenda. 1997. 'Employment Conditions for Nurses in Australia During World War II.' In *Nursing History*

and the Politics of Welfare, ed. Anne Marie Rafferty, Jane Robinson and Ruth Elkan. London and New York: Routledge, 192.

48. Bleakley, 'Memorandum'; Cilento to Ryan, September 29, 1939 and Ryan to Cilento, October 9, 1939. All in (1149, Box 57, Folder 925), Townsville Catholic Archives (TCA).
49. Queensland Department of Health and Home Affairs. c. 1937. *What Is Their Destiny?* Brisbane: Government Printing Press.
50. Ibid.
51. Hanlon, E.M. 'Memo: Fantome Island Leprosarium,' March 18, 1940 (Director of Native Affairs Office, 4513/1940, Batch file, Item ID ITM 717220), QSA.
52. Cilento to Ryan, October 19, 1939 (1149, Box 57, Folder 925), TCA.
53. Fisher, Fedora Gould. 1994. *Raphael Cilento: A Biography*. St. Lucia: University of Queensland Press, 4, 301–302.
54. Cilento to Ryan, December 8, 1939 (1149, Box 57, Folder 925), TCA.
55. Carey, Hilary M. 1998. 'Subordination, Invisibility and Chosen Work: Missionary Nuns and Australian Aborigines c.1900–1949.' *Australian Feminist Studie,* 13 (28), 257.
56. Cilento to Ryan, October 19, 1939 (1149, Box 57, Folder 925), TCA.
57. 'Vacancies for Settlement.' *Townsville Daily Bulletin*, March 13, 1940, 1.
58. Sisters of Our Lady Help of Christians (Australia). c. 1942. *Constitutions of the Congregation of the Sisters of the B.V.M. Under the Title of Help of Christians or the Sisters of Our Lady Help of Christians*. Manly: Sisters of Our Lady Help of Christians, Chapter 1, 4(b).
59. Deputy Director, Department of Native Affairs to Northern Territory Administrator, April 28, 1942 (A1928, 715/38 SECTION 1), NAA.
60. Kettle, Ellen. 1982. *A History of Channel Island in Darwin Harbour*. Darwin: The Author, 5.
61. Kirkland, Bruce. Report of Senior Medical Officer, June 4, 1942 (A431, 1950/3597), NAA.
62. Deputy Director, Medical Services, Northern Territory Forces to Director-General, Medical Services, January 23, 1943 (A1928, 715/38 SECTION 1), NAA.
63. Cumpston to Secretary, Department of the Army, February 22, 1943 (A1928, 715/38 SECTION 1), NAA.
64. Flynn, Reverend Frank. 1943. 'Channel Island Leper Station.' *The Annals of Our Lady of the Sacred Heart*. October 1, 183; Bryant, Sister Campion. n.d. 'Brief Biographies of OLSH Sisters who worked on Channel Island and East Arm, Northern Territory.' Daughters of Our Lady of the Sacred Heart Archives, Kensington, New South Wales (DOLSHK).
65. Cumpston to Minister, April 22, 1949 (A1658, 756/11/3 SECTION 1), NAA.

66. Venard, Mary. 1966. *The Designs of his Heart: Marie Louise Hartzer and the Congregation of the Daughters of Our Lady of the Sacred Heart.* Cork: The Mercier Press, 97, 144.
67. DOLSH Constitution, 1881, quoted in ibid., 160.
68. MacGinley, *A Dynamic of Hope*, 201, 259.
69. Venard, Mary. 1974. *The History of the Australian Province of the Daughters of Our Lady of the Sacred Heart.* Kensington: Daughters of Our Lady of the Sacred Heart, 1974, 136, 138.
70. Daughters of Our Lady of the Sacred Heart. 1928. *Constitutions of the Daughters of Our Lady of the Sacred Heart.* Westmead: Boys' Home, 6.
71. Ibid., 'Supplement to Rules: Relations with the Natives.'
72. Thomson, Ann. 1988. *NT Dreaming: The Story of the Catholic Church in the Northern Territory.* Darwin: Catholic Education Office, 44.
73. Carroll, Sister Benedicta. Interview with author. Typed transcript. Recorded at DOLSH Convent, Kensington, New South Wales, September 9, 2008.
74. Whelan, Sister Marion. Interview with author. Typed transcript. Recorded at DOLSH Convent, Kensington, New South Wales, August 12, 2008.
75. 'Helene May Cresp' (biography, no author), n.d., DOLSHK.
76. Moroney, Sister Angela SJG. 1977. Reminiscences (2.1A) SSJGB; Daly, Sister Alphonsus. 1986. *Healing Hands: memories and milestones of the Derby Leprosarium.* Perth: Health Department of Western Australia; Murnane, 'A Chaplet of Dolours.'
77. Carey, 'Subordination, Invisibility and Chosen Work,' 262.
78. Carroll, Interview with author; "Sister Jeanne" (name withheld). Interview with author. Typed transcript. Recorded at DOLSH Convent, Kensington, New South Wales. August 18, 2008.
79. *Constitutions of the Daughters of Our Lady of the Sacred Heart*, 1928, 6.
80. *The Australasian Catholic Directory.* Sydney: Australasian Catholic Directory, 1940, 507; O'Brien, Anne. 2005. *God's Willing Workers: Women and Religion in Australia.* Sydney: University of New South Wales Press, 164.
81. Murnane, *My Life as A Sister of St John of God*, 4; Daly, *Healing Hands.*
82. Whelan, Interview with author.
83. Reed, Margaret, 'Interview with Sister Mary Molloy—Palm and Fantome Island.' Franciscan Missionaries of Mary Archives, Summer Hill, New South Wales; Moroney, 'Reminiscences.'
84. Moroney, 'Reminiscences.'
85. *Australian Catholic Truth Society Record* 233. May 26, 1941; Eldridge, John. 1942. 'An Island Lazaret: The Story of an Heroic Missionary Enterprise.' *The Annals.* 2 February, 41–42; Flynn, 'Channel Island Leper Station'; Hennessy, J.J. c. 1949. *Missionary Sisters in Australia?* Kimberley: Sisters of St John of God.

86. O'Brien, *God's Willing Workers*, 122–123; de Vries, Susanna. 2010. 'Heroic Australian Women in War.' In *The Complete Book of Heroic Australian Women*, ed. Susanna de Vries. Pymble: HarperCollins, 308–310.
87. Turner, Naomi. 1988. *Which Seeds Shall Grow? Men and Women in Religious Life*. Melbourne: Collins Dove, 120.
88. Venard, *History of the Australian Province*, 169.

CHAPTER 5

The Leprosaria and Nursing Practice 1937–c.1950

Beginning work at the three different leprosaria—Fantome and Channel Islands and Derby—Sister nurses carried considerable expectations: to perform government health roles and the Church's mission mandate, not to mention their own spiritual ideals. The words of the Queensland Sisters' Superior, Mother Ignatius to the Bishop Ryan of Townsville indicate the hopes that underpinned the Sisters work: "Dr Cilento has great plans for a 'model' establishment at Fantome: please God the Sisters will do their part."[1] This chapter explores the first encounters between the Sisters and patients by explaining the backgrounds of the patients, their circumstances on arrival and conditions within the institutions, including staff. It then explores nursing care and medical treatments. It argues, counter to current historiography, that the engaging of Sister nurses by governments, rather than lay staff, was not a compromise on care. The appointed Sisters were fully trained and qualified nursing Sisters, most with midwifery qualifications and training in leprosy treatment. Although efficacious drugs were not introduced until the late 1940s, nursing before this era relieved symptoms, prevented or managed other conditions, and facilitated safe childbirth. Sisters and doctors persisted with new and existing therapies with hope and faith, despite disappointing results.

C. Robson, *Missionary Women, Leprosy and Indigenous Australians, 1936–1986*, https://doi.org/10.1007/978-3-031-05796-0_5

The Leprosaria and the Patients

Most patients at the leprosaria were Indigenous Australians, but within each institution, there were people from different regions, cultural and language groups, and individual backgrounds. When the Sisters arrived at Derby leprosarium in 1937, ninety patients were full or part-descent Indigenous from the Western Kimberley, including sixteen from Beagle Bay Mission, and several others from various cattle stations. Increasingly, more people were found in the East Kimberley at places such as Wyndham and Turkey Creek and at northern missions including Kunmunya and Kalumburu.[2] From 1940, some of the Western Australian patients who had been sent to Channel Island before the Derby Leprosarium was built also returned. Channel Island had 62 patients in 1943, including four European men. About half of the patients were from the mission stations at Port Keats, Roper River, Oenpelli and the Tiwi Islands; some were from scattered regions of Arnhem Land; and others from cattle stations, including Victoria Downs and Wave Hill.[3] The Fantome Island leprosarium, stated to be for 'coloured lepers' took all non-European patients from Peel Island leprosarium, among whom were people from the Mapoon mission in Cape York, and some originally from the Palm Island government settlement, making up the total of about 75 in 1940 when the OLHC Sisters arrived. Others admitted to this leprosarium were Torres Strait Islanders and Queenslanders with Pacific Islander heritage. Administratively, in Queensland, these groups, being dark-skinned, were classified as 'Aboriginal.'[4] A small proportion of the patients were children, some separated from their parents, and others, in the company of parents or other family members, who also suffered from the disease. Leprosy was common within families, but was not hereditary.

Invariably, these people arrived at the leprosarium under extremely distressing circumstances. Until at least the late 1940s, 'leper patrols', conducted in both states and the Northern Territory, routinely involved surprise raids by police or patrol officers on camps, after which 'suspects' would be rounded up, their necks chained, and forced to walk the long journey to the nearest holding compound until road, sea, or rail transport could be arranged. Others were identified at missions, schools, and pastoral stations, and brought in on the back of utility trucks, in 'leper' train carriages, or in the heaving holds of coastal luggers.[5] As a result of the patrols, Indigenous people became wary and frightened of police, white health workers and, in the Northern Territory, the patrol officers, referred to by one Channel Island patient as the man "who used to come 'round trying to grab us."[6] Indigenous people hid in the bush at any hint of their impending presence. They had seen their relatives being taken away to the leprosarium, never to return—they feared the same for themselves.

From the point of view of leprosy patients, they were better off with their own families and on their own land, especially if they were very ill. They were not the abandoned who needed rescuing, as the missionaries portrayed them. John Hargrave, a leprosy specialist who, for thirty years from the 1950s, treated Northern Territory Indigenous people stated,

> Whatever their feelings, whatever their beliefs, whatever their attitudes, Aborigines never shun a leprosy patient. They care for him in the camp. Far better, they believe, that he die in his own country deformed and disabled, than that he be taken away to die away from his totemic waterhole.[7]

As leprosarium patients, Indigenous people severed contact with their families, sometimes permanently. Only from the 1950s were they permitted adult visitors but even then, the long distances limited or prevented visits for some families. On the other hand, because leprosy was passed through families and communities, many patients knew or were related to others, an awful yet mitigating circumstance.[8] The concentration of people from different tribal groups led to tension and sometimes violence yet it also sometimes fostered unusual affiliations in which friendships developed, and cultural and linguistic exchange took place (Fig. 5.1).

The leprosaria were planned as semi self-sufficient villages, similar to Indigenous mission settlements or the Peel Island leprosarium in southern Queensland. The design and placement of the buildings reflected sanitary objectives of state health authorities and racial paradigms, as well as tight budgetary constraints. Men and women were housed in separate sections and fenced off. Young women and children, also separated according to gender, were accommodated in dormitory-style housing.[9] Sexual segregation was a government health policy in line with current international practices for the purpose of preventing reproduction and the infecting of the newborn with the disease through parental contact.[10] Nevertheless, attempts at keeping the sexes apart repeatedly failed.

At each leprosarium, most adults lived in clustered small huts, each designed for two to four people. The rationale for this arrangement was

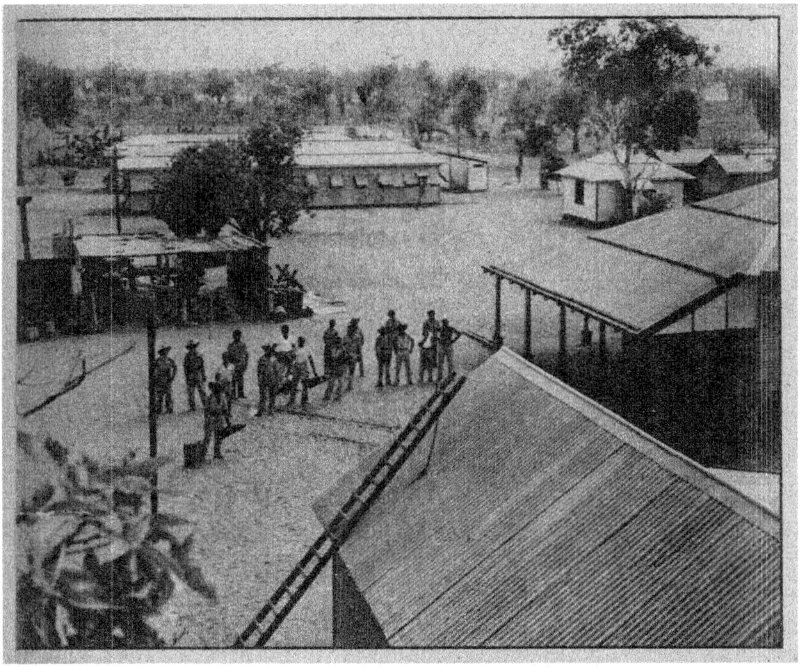

Fig. 5.1 Work sheds, hospital, and dormitories at Derby Leprosarium 1947 (*Pix*, September 13, 1947, 5)

to prevent cramped living conditions which were believed to encourage the spread of leprosy. But as patient numbers increased in the 1940s, the huts became overcrowded and, after years of delay and protest, extra accommodation was supplied. In Derby, this upgrade consisted of a pair of long dormitory-style buildings, one each for the men and women. Most huts were of primitive construction, having wooden frames with walls of either galvanised iron or fibrocement, concrete slab floors, and with little furniture other than a bed. They offered scarce respite from the severe heat and heavy rains of the northern Australian wet seasons. Mostly, they served as sleeping quarters since, for much of the day, the patients engaged in activities that took them either outdoors or into one of the common buildings reserved for dining, bathing, treatment, recreation, and school. Residents who were acutely ill or non-ambulatory stayed in the leprosarium hospitals which were divided into female and male wards.[11]

This form of accommodation was designed with Indigenous patients in mind, the justification being that they had previously not been accustomed to dwellings of any higher standard.[12] The few patients of Channel Island and Derby who were European or mainly of European descent had more private quarters, set apart from the main settlement. At Channel Island, two male European patients built an "iron shack" for themselves near the beach, away from the main settlement, and at Derby, three part-descent sisters were given a multi-roomed cottage near the staff quarters.[13] The detention of people of predominantly European heritage in the leprosaria did not sit well in the minds of government doctors and other officials and the prospect of more such admissions to Derby prompted District Medical Officer, A.R. Haynes, to protest, "This institution is only a [sic] Aboriginal hospital or leprosarium...You could not take either the quadroon men or women and dump them in a blackfellow camp."[14] On Fantome Island, no such official sympathy was expressed since skin colour, rather than ethnicity, defined all patients as 'Aboriginal.' Thus, third-generation Melanesians from south-eastern Queensland country towns were considered as suited to the primitive dwellings as were Indigenous Australians.

On the arrival of the Sisters at the newer facilities at Fantome Island and Derby, agricultural development was begun with bright-eyed optimism in the purchase of livestock and vegetable seeds, and the construction of accessories such as wells, bakehouses, and windmills. Initially, supplies were shipped in until the regular production of foodstuffs could begin. It became evident, however, that the water supply would not be adequate for self-sufficiency. The long dry weather spells and the absence of natural waterways that characterised the sites of all three institutions led to the failure of food crops and the death, or lack of productivity, of farm animals. Goats did not produce enough milk at Fantome Island and the sheep at Derby perished. At times, there was barely enough water for washing. Until after World War II, the leprosarium communities continued to be highly dependent upon the transport of almost all their needs from town, but poor communication, wartime interruptions, and hazardous weather conditions made deliveries unreliable. Without refrigeration and in such extreme heat, meat had to be consumed immediately, and then there would be no more for long periods.[15] Consequently, patients went without fresh fruit, meat, vegetables, and water, all of which were stipulated by leprosarium planners as essential for their well-being and recovery. To survive, the communities had to lean on their own or the Sisters' resources.

The degree of responsibility officially delegated to the Sisters varied across the institutions and depended to some extent on the authority granted to lay administrative staff. Government authorities believed that male superintendents were essential for the Sisters' protection, to regulate the behaviour of the male patients, and to run the administration generally. In Western Australia, authorities emphasised that the Sisters were only to perform nursing duties, and that the senior Sister, Mother Gertrude, was not to be accorded the title of 'matron.'[16] A superintendent and his wife were employed as administrators and, although Mother Gertrude tried to assume responsibility for requisitioning the patients' clothes, medicines, and food, she was informed that she would have to liaise over these issues through the superintendent.

At Fantome Island, Mother Peter was designated 'matron' and given charge of the general care and welfare of the patients, the domestic affairs of the institution, the discipline of the patients, and the issue of drugs and medical supplies, stores, clothing, bedding and linen. In this capacity, she was still subject to a superintendent's authority. Frank Julian, however, who held this position, also oversaw the lock hospital at the opposite end of the island so had little time for the leprosarium.[17] Furthermore, he vacated the position in 1947 and was not replaced.

The Daughters of Our Lady of the Sacred Heart (DOLSH) Sisters arrived at Channel Island in 1943, with the re-establishment of the leprosarium during the military occupation of the Northern Territory. Surviving patients, who had been released the year before and told to evacuate to the mainland, had been brought back. Mother Campion recalled that the dangers of air raids remained, and the rush to get everyone into shelters.

> From Channel Island I could turn in my bed and look towards Darwin Harbour. Should it be in darkness then we knew the enemy was near. Time and time again we heard planes roar over us and bombs bursting and watched dog fights in the sky and also watched blazing planes falling.[18]

Few civilian women were permitted in the Darwin area at this time but concerns about female fragility in a war zone appeared not to apply to religious Sisters. Their reputation for self-sacrifice, performed in the service of God, somehow qualified them for equally challenging work in the service of their country—in this case, custodians of leprosy patients deemed dangerous to the American soldiers in the Territory. They were expected to cope with the threat of enemy attack, and, perhaps, for them, it was no worse than the weather extremes, dangerous fauna, primitive living conditions and the infectious diseases that came their way as missionaries. Their role in defending the nation set them apart from other women who, by becoming mothers, were valued as nation-builders in that period.[19]

For Darwin priest, William Henschke, however, the Sisters' safety was a concern. He admired their nonchalance as they soldiered on in the clinic while bombs raged outside, but, refusing to leave them alone, installed himself in an old garage until a male superintendent could be appointed. "...Sisters like a man near at hand and they feel they have a protector, especially in these settled [sic] times", he claimed to his Provincial Superior, evidently overlooking the male patients for this role.[20] He feared the sexual predations of the enemy, who he asserted, "have no respect for the nuns or girls."[21]

With few civilians remaining in Darwin, there was little choice but to appoint a missionary to the role of male superintendent. The Catholic bishop of Darwin, Francis Xavier Gsell, arranged for a Brother of his own order, the MSC, to take the position. Extensive testimony suggests that, for the six years he spent there, Brother McCarthy quietly performed his manual duties, such as managing the stores, and was friendly towards the patients, but did little to discipline the patients, as was expected.[22] The Sisters, then, like their Fantome Island counterparts, were left with a great deal of responsibility in the areas of discipline and administration.

The Derby Sisters were also thrust into danger and forced to rely on their own resources and those of the patients, when air raids began in the Kimberley in early 1942. Although urged to evacuate by plane and leave the patients, Mother Gertrude refused and took to the bush with three Sisters and the patients. With the help of the stronger patients, they brought with them food and supplies, set up a makeshift clinic and living quarters, and waited it out for several weeks. When the leprosarium superintendent drove past and offered them another chance of evacuation, the Sisters again refused to leave the patients. Sister Peter Evans, a young novice, described the experience in a letter to her mother:

> During February after Darwin had been bombed, things began to liven up here…Mother told me to finish up and go for Sister who was in the camps as we had to get into our trenches, for Wyndham had been raided and Broome was even then being raided and we would be next.[23]

Exchanging their glary white habits for dark cloaks, hiding in the long grass, drinking water "from a small billabong where all the lepers were dipping their pannikins and washing themselves" and, finally, facing a food shortage due to the absence of sea transport, were all described by Evans with a note of bravado.[24]

Mother Gertrude almost certainly thought the patients would die if left to fend for themselves. She also, by this time, had longstanding connections with some, especially those who had been part of the Beagle Bay Mission where she had also worked. She would have been unaware of the release into the bush of the Channel Island patients at the same time, including some people who had been sent up from Beagle Bay under the old policy, like Gregory Howard. These incidents highlight the dependence Indigenous people had on missions and leprosaria for the provision of food and shelter. The extent to which nursing care also contributed to their survival cannot be determined. We might speculate about the patients who did not accompany Mother Gertrude into hiding, but disappeared and were mostly never heard of again. They may not have had institutional backgrounds and been capable of living off the land or sea, and perhaps they were not sick patients and therefore not reliant on nursing care. Could they have been better off with their freedom? Perhaps, but it was not easy to survive in unfamiliar country, nor to find one's way home across vast unknown territory.

Nursing and Medical Care

"…Attend to sores, treat other diseases, give injections twice weekly, take temperatures…" was the brief given to the Derby sisters when they began work at the leprosarium in 1937; instructions to sisters at the other institutions were similar.[25] But the scope of their nursing roles was much more extensive and the tasks more challenging than these lists suggest. The deficiencies and particular demands of these far-flung under-resourced institutions meant that often unassigned and unexpected responsibilities fell to the nursing staff. As patient numbers increased and therapeutics changed over the years, the nursing became more labour-intensive and complex, with a diversification of their tasks. Yet, existing histories have labelled the nursing work of the sisters as "rudimentary" and prone to error. Their qualifications have been downgraded, with the Sisters being described as "untrained" and "nuns instead of nurses", as if these categories were mutually exclusive.[26] The evidence put forward in this chapter suggests otherwise.

From the beginning of the Catholic Sisters' association with the three leprosaria in northern Australia—Derby and Channel and Fantome Islands—every nurse on staff was fully trained in accredited hospitals, bringing their qualifications in line with those of lay registered nursing sisters. Second, at each institution, at least one, but more commonly, several, were double or triple certificated nurses, qualifying them for maternity and mothercraft nursing.[27] In addition to basic nursing, the Sisters acquired specific knowledge of leprosy nursing and diagnostic techniques. Before the first group of Sisters began at Fantome Island, they were trained by medical officer, D.W. Johnson, at Peel Island and at the government laboratory in Brisbane by Raphael Cilento, expert in tropical diseases and Queensland Director-general of Health and Medical Services. As well as leprosy nursing, they were taught "laboratory work and staining methods, instruction in the pulling of teeth and dispensing."[28] Cilento assured the Bishop of Townsville that "they will go up with a very much better knowledge of the work than any other nursing sisters have had when they commenced work amongst lepers in this country."[29] The Sisters "devoured" medical texts on leprosy and the Queensland sisters underwent courses in tropical medicine at Sydney University.[30] Their appointment at Fantome was arranged well in advance, giving enough time to prepare them, whereas the Sisters of Derby and Channel Island, having little notice of their impending assignments, received on-site instruction from medical officers and some had previous experience on the missions. The first Sisters at Derby were told by their Provincial Superior "to study books on leprosy" whenever they had free time.[31] Several Sisters underwent specialist courses after the Second World War, such as Mother Alphonsus Daly of the Derby leprosarium, who studied tropical medicine at Sydney University.[32] Some senior Sisters remained nursing at the leprosaria for many years, accumulating extensive experience, including Daly, described by the Commissioner of Health in 1954 as "an authority on leprosy beyond the normal sphere of a nursing Sister."[33]

The engagement of full-time medical officers, knowledgeable in leprosy medicine, had been considered essential in doctors' visions of the new leprosaria at Derby and Fantome Island as "modern and up-to-date treatment centres."[34] But soon after both facilities opened, the difficulties of obtaining medical staff for this work became clear. It was during Australia's involvement in World War II that Fantome Island opened. The doctor poised to take the medical superintendent's position joined the navy in 1940 and was not replaced. For Derby, no suitable applicants, including from among medical missionaries, could be found.[35] Senior state officials in both Queensland and Western Australia, faced with the costs and shortages in available personnel became easily persuaded that "the treatment of leprosy is more or less routine" and that "the Sisters carry out the treatment necessary."[36] The position of a full-time doctor was therefore seen as redundant, and as the case had been for Channel Island since its establishment in 1931, medical work at the leprosaria became part of the overall duties of local medical officers, supplemented by the occasional visits of specialists.[37] This system never changed in the two states, despite the growing complexity of treatment regimens and a threefold increase in patients at Derby by the early 1950s. Only in the Northern Territory, after the relocation of the leprosarium to the mainland, was a full-time doctor eventually employed in the late 1950s. In contrast, at the European leprosarium on Peel Island a full-time medical officer was employed from 1944.[38]

As well as losing its medical officer, Fantome Island lost the services of Graham Croll, the leprosy research officer funded by a grant from the National Health and Medical Research Council (NHMRC) in 1939, who resigned in the same year, due to illness. In addition to inspection tours of northern Queensland, Croll was to have conducted research and provided ongoing training to the nursing staff on Fantome Island, along with the medical officer. None of these tasks became possible then, or at any other stage. Cilento, furious with medical attendance reduced to the cursory visits of the elderly and inexperienced Palm Island medical officer, proclaimed, "Until a solution is found…, medical work at Fantome Island will be entirely unsatisfactory and constantly subject to justifiable criticism."[39]

The corresponding NHMRC investigation officer for the north-west of Western Australia was Louis A. Musso who, on expiry of the grant in 1941, became medical officer of the Western Australian Department of Aborigines until 1947. As part of these roles, Musso spent a considerable amount of time at the Derby leprosarium, training the Sisters in aspects of testing and treatment, tailoring therapies to each patient, improving their diets, and monitoring outcomes.[40] In 1945, he instituted the policy of admitting only those showing bacteriological evidence of the disease (apart from some exceptional cases), rather than, as in other leprosaria, positive clinical signs being sufficient cause. As a consequence of his influence, Derby was the only Indigenous leprosarium to discharge significant numbers of patients before the early 1950s, some due to the arrest of their disease and others, found to have the less infectious form of the disease, deemed unnecessarily detained.[41]

In the 1930s and 1940s, most leprologists recommended chaulmoogra oil as treatment for leprosy, believing that, combined with improved nutrition, housing, and exercise, it was capable of lessening the effects of leprosy or, at best, arresting the disease.[42] However, it was not a cure, as some nurses, doctors and patients realised, and improvements in patients' conditions were increasingly being explained by the occasional tendency of the disease to spontaneously resolve, rather than resulting from chaulmoogra therapy. But it was the only agent medicine could offer. Medical officers also prescribed specific diets for all patients, but their uptake by health departments, at least for Indigenous patients, was patchy, and severely interrupted by wartime transport and supply problems. Added to the poor housing, the co-existence of other illnesses and the emotional trauma of separation from home and family, the outlook for patients was indeed grim and it would hardly be a surprise if they did not benefit from the medication given. What slender hope was held for their cure at the outset of treatment must surely have diminished even further as patients passed rapidly away, and survival itself remained a tenuous goal. By 1945, close to 30% of patients had died at Derby and 37% at Fantome Island. Comparable figures for Channel Island are unavailable; for the period 1932–1938, approximately 34% died.[43]

Yet, the Sisters remained hopeful, diligent, and inventive, if not always expecting a cure, at least to palliate. Sister Angela, looking back on her nursing work at Derby in the early 1940s, remembered,

> Every evening Mother gathered all the Catholics and anyone else who wanted to come for rosary and novena for the request of a cure for leprosy. Dr Musso urged them to keep up the novenas. He said, 'one day a cure will come and when it does come it will be a quick one.[44]

Until the late 1940s, the Sisters administered chaulmoogra oil, either orally or by injection, usually twice weekly. It was a thick, oily substance that Mother Alphonsus remembered heating on a flame over a kerosene stove before injecting into patients' limbs or the edges of their skin lesions.[45] The pain would have been excruciating. At Channel Island, Sister Benedicta poured the oil into capsules for swallowing, but it still made patients feel ill and so unwilling to take it, and she recalled how some "put it behind their ear or somewhere and drank the water."[46] Side-effects ranged from nausea, vomiting and fever to liver and blood toxicities. So, it was not only to find more efficacious substances, but to improve compliance that the search for other drugs was seen as vital. For the patients, this meant trials with new drugs were a constant part of life in the leprosarium.

Each month, the Sisters tested for the leprosy bacillus. Serum (known as 'smears') from the tissue of the patients' ear lobes, nose and eyebrows was extracted, stained and examined under the microscope for the presence of the bacteria. Results were recorded along with clinical observations and used to chart the course of the disease in each patient. Smear tests detected the infectivity of the patient and, taken in a continued series over months and years, revealed the course of the disease in the individual. An unbroken set of negative smears over periods that varied between twelve and twenty-four months, depending on medical opinion at particular times, along with clinical improvement over two years, was evidence of the arrest of the disease.[47]

A large part of the Sisters' days, and, sometimes, nights, was occupied with managing and trying to ameliorate the multifarious and sometimes serious conditions and complications induced by the disease and the distressing and painful reactions many experienced to leprosy medication. Twice daily, they attended to the routine clinical procedures: giving out medication for various conditions, washing and bandaging the patients' lesions, paring ulcers, and applying caustics. At other times, they were in the dispensary, mixing solutions and compresses, or performing dental extractions. If amputations or other medical procedures were required, they assisted and then took charge of the patient's recovery (Fig. 5.2).[48]

The Sisters also devised their own ways to improve the patients' health. Formal physiotherapy and occupational therapy regimes were not incorporated into the leprosaria until at least the 1960s (and not at all in

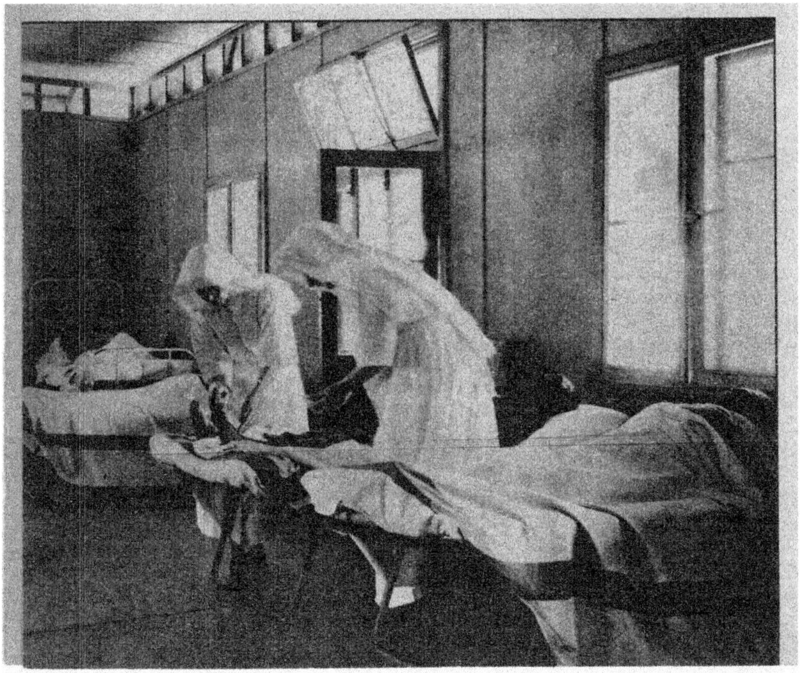

Fig. 5.2 Sister attending to hospital patient, Derby Leprosarium 1947 (*Pix*, September 13, 1947, 5)

the case of Fantome Island) although the benefit of physical exercise to the leprosy patient's physical and mental condition was appreciated by leprologists at least as far back as the interwar period. In particular, the importance of exercising limbs to prevent or at least minimise the development of deformities, such as nerve contractures, and a range of other debilitating conditions associated with leprosy, has long been recognised. At Derby, patients lined up each day in separate groups of men and women, and were taken through their exercises. At all leprosaria, sports events were organised, including football matches for both sexes. Hands and fingers were exercised with painting, sculpting, and playing musical instruments (see Chapter 6) and women spun, weaved, knitted, and sewed (Fig. 5.3).[49]

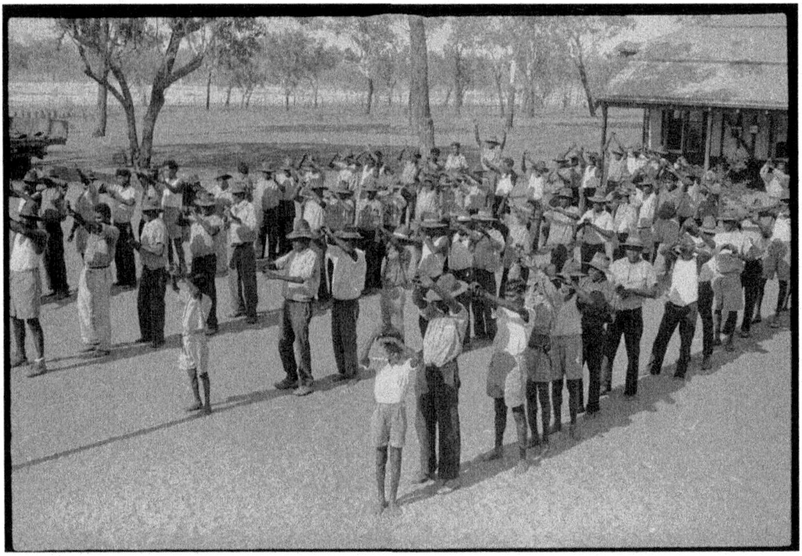

Fig. 5.3 'Daily Exercise Class, Derby Leprosarium 1948' (Stuart Gore Collection, State Library of Western Australia)

Enduring images cast from first-hand accounts depict nights spent by these earlier Sisters hovering over patients with kerosene lamps, keeping fevers down and easing pains, and in the less hopeful cases, providing comfort.[50] As intended, they convey the heroism, skill, and dedication of the nurses but, considering they are images from the mid-twentieth century, they also highlight the grave inadequacies of the leprosaria as medical institutions. Electricity was not supplied to Fantome Island until 1953; in emergencies, staff lit a fire to attract the attention of the Palm Islanders and then waited long hours for assistance. When a dangerously premature birth took place on Channel Island in 1952, one of the patients rowed the eight miles to the mainland to bring back a doctor. Nevertheless, the newborn child remained in the care of the leprosarium Sisters until its health improved, reportedly using a humidicrib fashioned by Brother Lilwall, the superintendent (Fig. 5.4).[51]

The Sisters took precautions to avoid contracting leprosy from the patients. A few months after the Derby Sisters began their work, the SSJG

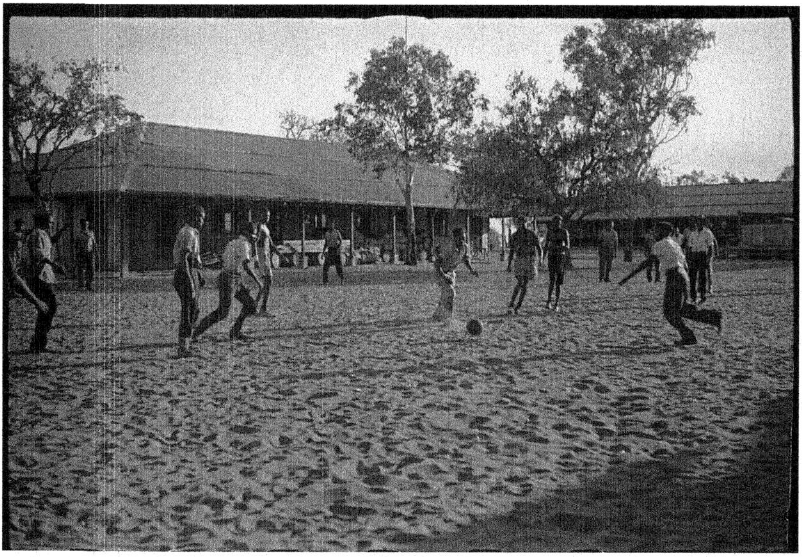

Fig. 5.4 'Barefoot Football Derby Leprosarium 1948' (Stuart Gore Collection, State Library of WA)

Kimberley Superior, Mother Margaret, informed them of sanitation practices they were to follow. Before beginning work, they were to change out of the veils, gowns, and shoes they had put on in the convent into another set kept in a hospital cupboard, and the convent clothes were to be stored in a separate compartment. When finished for the day, they were to reverse the process. The Sisters had to gargle after close contact with the patients, and "everything made by them must be disinfected before being used by the Sisters."[52] This last instruction refers to the dressmaking and carpentry done by the patients.

New technology and new drugs, whenever available, were taken up with enthusiasm by the Sisters. Ultraviolet ray treatment at Derby was one example that eventually proved of limited benefit. Mother Alphonsus devised her own system of classifying the leprosy bacilli observed with the microscope to help identify patients' progress, well before the formal 'Morphological Index' was invented.[53] In 1946, Sister Michaeline, the second Channel Island matron, heard of a new drug called Promin, hailed as a great success at overseas leprosaria, and she immediately approached the health department for supplies.[54] Promin belonged to the sulphones class of drugs. It was highly toxic and only available as an injection, therefore careful administration and continual monitoring of its effects were essential. Mother Michaeline was advised that as treatment required full-time medical supervision, it could not be supplied to Indigenous patients.[55] At Peel Island leprosarium where a doctor was permanently stationed, Promin treatment began the next year but even here, only 1/3 of the patients could be treated due to medical staff shortages. In 1948, administration of sulphones finally began at all three leprosaria for Indigenous patients with the introduction of Sulphetrone, given orally.[56]

* * *

Despite the obvious tensions between forcible incarceration and good care, the leprosaria were envisaged by doctors and government departments as modern institutions with the necessary medical and nursing care, diet, and conditions. However, in many respects these hopes were dashed. The remoteness of the institutions—the very reason their sites were chosen—obstructed medical oversight and the provision of basic supplies. The situation was exacerbated with the outbreak of World War II. Contact was cut off with the bombing of Darwin and the Kimberley coastline, doctors enlisted, and widespread shortages of supplies such as food and building materials until the late 1940s impacted on the leprosaria. Consequently, Sisters and patients were forced to rely on their own resources to a large degree. Nevertheless, medical and nursing care within these constraints continued.

Notes

1. Murnane, Mother Ignatius to Bishop Hugh Ryan, 31 December 1939 (1149, Box 57, Folder 925), Townsville Cathedral Archives (TCA).
2. Western Australian Department of Native Affairs. 1937. *Annual Report of the Commissioner of Native Affairs for* the Year Ending 30 June 1937. Perth: Government Printer, 9–11; Davidson, W.S. 1978. *Havens of Refuge: A History of Leprosy in Western Australia*. Perth: University of Western Australia Press for the Public Health Department, 65–78.

3. Cumpston, J.H.L. to Secretary, Relatives and Friends Assocation, January 10, 1952 (A1658, 258/1/1 PART 1), National Archives of Australia (NAA); Nominal Roll, April 12, 1949 (F1 1952/526), NAA.
4. Rowley, C.D. 1970. *The Destruction of Aboriginal Society: Aboriginal Policy and Practice*, volume one. Canberra: Australian National University Press, 363.
5. Mowaljarlai, David. 2001. *Yorro: Everything Standing Up Alive: Spirit of the Kimberley*. Broome: Magabala Books, 117–119; Former patient "A" (name withheld). Interview with Christine Choo, 1992, sound recording, State Library of Western Australia; Saunders, Suzanne, 1989. *'A Suitable Island Site': Leprosy in the Northern Territory and the Channel Island Leprosarium 1880–1955*. Darwin: Historical Society of the Northern Territory, 46–48.
6. Kerinaiua, Philomena. c. 2002. 'Philomena's Story.' In *So Far From Home: Oral Histories of the Stolen Generations*, ed. Lana Quall. Katherine: Diwurruwurru-jaru Aboriginal Corporation, 28.
7. Hargrave, J.C. 1975. Leprosy in the Northern Territory of Australia: with Particular Reference to the Aborigines of Arnhem Land and the Arid Regions of the Northern Territory. M.D. diss., University of Sydney, 253–254.
8. Eggmolesse, Joe (former patient) in Gilligan, Sean and Adrian Strong. 2011. 'Fantome Island.' Videorecording. Australian Capital Territory: Ronin Films.
9. Huelin, Frederick (Under-Secretary), 'Memo-Derby Leprosarium,' 7 July 1937 (Public Health Department, 1935/0251, Cons 1003), State Records Office Western Australia (SROWA); 'Report of Investigating Committee' (Channel Island), November 19, 1946, 3 (A1928, 715/38/1 SECTION 3), NAA; Our Lady Help of Christians. 'Monthly Journal, Fantome Island,' March 1941 (1144, Box 57, Folder 920), TCA.
10. Rogers, Leonard and Ernest Muir. 1946. *Leprosy*, third edition. Baltimore: The Williams and Wilkins Co., 129–131.
11. Trigg, Memo, August 12, 1935 (PHD, 1935/0251, Cons 1003), SROWA; 'Report of investigating committee, November 19, 1946, 3 (A1928, 715/38/1 SECTION 3), NAA; Gabriel, Morgan. 'Report on Visit to Fantome Island-April 1953,' 3 (Director of Native Affairs Office, 3A/153, Correspondence, Aboriginal and Torres Strait Islander, ITM505017), QSA; Parsons, Meg. 2008. Spaces of Disease: the Creation and Management of Aboriginal Health and Disease in Queensland 1900–1970. Ph.D. diss., University of Sydney, 346–348.
12. Carroll, Sister Benedicta OLSH. Interview with author. Typed transcript. Recorded at Kensington, New South Wales, September 9, 2008.

13. 'Report of Investigating Committee' (A1928, 715/38/1 SECTION 3), NAA; Assistant Under Secretary, Memo, c.1941 (PHD, 1940/0390, Cons 1003), SROWA.
14. Haynes, A.R. to Atkinson, Everitt (Commissioner of Public Health, Western Australia), April 29, 1941 (PHD, 1940/0390, Cons 1003), SROWA.
15. For descriptions of these conditions, see: Butler, Major A.J. (Australian Military Forces, Northern Territory Force), 'Channel Island,' December 14, 1944 (A1928, 715/38/1 SECTION 2), NAA; 'Report of the Investigating Committee,' 5–6 (A1928, 715/38/1 SECTION 3), NAA; Greene, Sister Gertrude to Atkinson, May 15, 1939 and Davis, Albert to Atkinson, May 13, 1937 (PHD, 1935/0251, Cons 1003), SROWA; Former patients "A" and "B" (names withheld). Interviews with Christine Choo, 1992, sound recordings, State Library of Western Australia; Lachance, Sister M. Marguerite. 'Fantome Island History.' Franciscan Missionaries of Mary Archives, Summer Hill, New South Wales (FMMS); Duford, Sister Paule, interview with Siobhan McHugh, *Siobhan McHugh Collection of Australian Social History*. Sound recording, 198–?, ORAL TRC 2761/5, National Library of Australia (NLA); Parsons, Spaces of Disease, 343–346.
16. Atkinson to Huelin, May 1939 (PHD, 1935/0251, Cons 1003), SROWA.
17. Under-Secretary to Minister, 'Fantome Leprosarium: Working Organisation,' May 13, 1940 (Director of Native Affairs Office, 4513/1940, Batch file, ID ITM717220), QSA.
18. Bryant, Sr Campion. n.d. 'Channel Island,' Memoirs, Daughters of Our Lady of the Sacred Heart Archives, Kensington (DOLSHK).
19. Riddett, Lyn A. 1991. 'Guarding Civilisation's Rim: The Australian Inland Mission Sisters in the Victoria River District 1922–1939.' *Journal of Australian Studies* 15 (30), 39.
20. Henschke, Fr William to Kerrins, Fr Joseph, April 29, 1943 (Provincial Correspondence, NT Darwin 1943), Missionaries of the Sacred Heart Archives Kensington (MSCK).
21. Henschke to Kerrins, February 1, 1942 (Prov Corr, NT Darwin 1942), MSCK.
22. 'Inquiry Re: Channel Island - Leper Station,' November 12, 1946 (A1928, 715/38/1 SECTION 3), NAA.
23. Evans, Sr Peter to her parents, April 1942 (2.9 M), Sisters of St John of God Archives, Broome (SSJGB).
24. Ibid.
25. Carmody, Mother Margaret to Huelin, August 3, 1937 (PHD, 1935/0251, Cons 1003), SROWA.

26. Edmond, Rod. 2006. *Leprosy and Empire: A Medical and Cultural History.* New York: Cambridge University Press, 167; Genever, Geoff. 2008. 'Queensland's Black Leper Colony.' *Queensland Review* 15 (2), 64; Parsons, Spaces of Disease, 336.
27. Whelan, Sister Marion OLSH. Interview with author. Typed transcript. Recorded at Kensington, New South Wales, August 12, 2008; Benedicta. Interview; Poidevin, Sister Camille SJG. Interview with author. Typed transcript. Recorded at Derby, Western Australia, November 17, 2008; "Sister Helen" OLSH (name withheld). Interview with author. Typed transcript. Recorded at Kensington, NSW, August 18, 2008; "Sr Jeanne" OLSH (name withheld). Interview with author. Typed transcript. Recorded at Kensington, New South Wales, August 18, 2008.
28. Cilento, Raphael to Ryan, Bishop Hugh, February 2, 1940 (1148, Box 57, Folder 924), TCA.
29. Ibid.
30. Ibid; Ignatius to Ryan, December 31,1939 and May 12, 1940 (1148, Box 57, Folder 924), TCA; MacGinley, M.R. 2010. *An Eloquent Witness: The Sisters of Our Lady Help of Christians.* Strathfield: St Pauls Publications, 100.
31. Mother Margaret. 'Suggestions About Alterations in the Convent,' July 28, 1937 (2.621), SSJGB.
32. 'The SJG Sisters in the Kimberley District N.W. Australia,' n.d. (2.60O), SSJGB.
33. 'Derby Leprosarium Staff Duties,' May 13, 1954 (E51, 1960/277), NAA.
34. Davis to Atkinson, September 14, 1936 (PHD, 1935/0732, Cons 1003), SROWA.
35. Atkinson to Davis, June 21, 1937 (PHD, 1935/0251, Cons 1003), SROWA.
36. Huelin, Frederick. 'Memorandum: Derby Leprosarium,' July 7, 1937 (PHD, 1935/0251, Cons 1003, SROWA); Coffey, J. to the Under-Secretary, 1940 (4513/1940, ITM717220), QSA.
37. Saunders, '*A Suitable Island Site*,' 36; 'Memorandum: Derby Leprosarium,' July 7, 1937 (PHD, 1935/0251, Cons 1003), SROWA; Under-Secretary to Minister, 'Fantome Leprosarium: Working Organisation,' May 13, 1940 (4513/1940, ITM717220), QSA.
38. Parsons, Spaces of Disease, 287.
39. Cilento to Under-Secretary, August 9, 1940 (4513/1940, ITM717220), QSA.
40. Davidson, *Havens of Refuge*, 79.
41. Musso, L.A. 'A General Review of the Cases of Leprosy from 1935 to October 1945,' February 15, 1946 (Department of Native Affairs, 1946/0392, Cons 993), SROWA. Between 1940 and 1950, over 200

patients were discharged from Derby, 32 from Channel Island and 9 from Fantome Island. See Musso, 'A General Review,' 5; Bateman, F.E.A. 1948. *Report on Survey of Native Affairs*. Perth: Government Printer, 20; Queensland Health and Medical Services Branch. 1964. *Annual Report on* the Health and Medical Services of the State of Queensland. Brisbane: The State, 14; Humphry, A.H. 1952. 'Leprosy Among Full-Blooded Aborigines.' *The Medical Journal of Australia* 17 (1), 570.

42. Rogers and Muir, Leprosy, 242–243; Musso, 'A General Review,' 5–6.
43. Musso, 'A General Review,' 5–6; Queensland Department of Health and Home Affairs, *Annual Report 1964*, 14; Saunders, '*A Suitable Island Site*,' 42.
44. Moroney, Sr Angela. Reminiscences (2.1A), SSJGB.
45. Daly, Sister Alphonus M. 1986. *Healing Hands: Memories and Milestones of the Derby Leprosarium*. Perth: Health Department of Western Australia, 1986.
46. Sr Benedicta, Interview with author.
47. Lachance, 'Fantome Island History'; *Leprosy in Northern Territory Aborigines*. Darwin: Northern Territory Medical Service, 1968, 26–27.
48. Lachance, 'Fantome Island History'; Moloney, Sister Anna FMM (formerly Sister Catherine OLHC), 'My Journey in Religious Life from 1935–1969,' FMMS.
49. Moonot, P., Ashwood, N. and D. Lockwood. 2005. 'Orthopaedic Complications of Leprosy.' *The Journal of Bone and Joint Surgery* 87 (10), 1329–1330; Hunn, Patricia M. 1971. 'Leprosy: Ancient Disease, Modern Challenge!' *Australian Journal of Physiotherapy* 3, September, 100; Gore, Stuart. 1951. 'Leper Colony.' *Walkabout*, November 1, 19; "John" (former patient, Fantome Island Leprosarium). Interview with author. 7 June 2011. Typed transcript. Location and name confidential.
50. Henschke to Kerrins, September 10, 1946 (Prov. Corr. N.T. Darwin 1946), MSCK; Moroney, 'Reminiscences'; Moloney, 'My Journey.'
51. Lachance, 'Fantome Island History'; '24 oz Baby Born to Leper.' *The Sunday Herald*, June 22, 1952, 1.
52. Mother Margaret. 'Suggestions About Alterations in the Convent,' July 28, 1937 (2.621), SSJGB.
53. Davidson, *Havens of Refuge*, 114.
54. Metcalfe, A.J. (Acting Commonwealth Director-General of Health) to McGlashan, John (Chief Medical Officer, Northern Territory), December 9, 1946 (A1928, 715/38/1 SECTION 3), NAA.
55. Reye, Eric. 'Leprosy in Queensland.' In Queensland Health and Medical Services Branch. 1947. *Annual Report on the Health and Medical Services of the State of Queensland for the year 1946–1947*. Brisbane: The State, 7; McGlashan to Promotion Manager, Parke Davis & Co. November 6, 1947 (A1928, 715/38/1 SECTION 3), NAA.

56. Queensland Health and Medical Services Branch, *Annual* Report 1946–1947, 7–8 and 1948–1949, 13; Dr Herz cited in Davidson, *Havens of Refuge*, 174; Parry, Suzanne. 2003. '"Of Vital Importance to the Community": The Control of Leprosy in the Northern Territory.' Health and History, 5 (1), 2; Humphry, 'Leprosy Among Full-Blooded Aborigines,' 73.

CHAPTER 6

Social, Cultural and Spiritual Life in the Leprosarium

The Sisters initiated or implemented a range of activities for Indigenous leprosarium patients aimed for their control and solace, and to assimilate them to Western Christian culture. To an extent, these activities recognised the despair and anger invoked by institutional restrictions and the prospect of lifelong incarceration and looked to prevent violence and abscondings that threatened public health goals and institutional harmony. For the Sisters, the solution was to socialise patients to an institutional model influenced by their own missionary ideals. They attempted to heal and train the bodies, souls, and minds of their patients; taught Western education, handcrafts, music, and dance; tried to instil Western notions of hygiene, morality, and respectability; and revealed a suffering Christ with whom patients might identify, as leprosy sufferers and members of a dispossessed race. Pleasure and creativity were pursued as cathartic, with concerts and parties or patients' traditional activities, such as dance, fishing, and handcrafts. Patients sometimes resisted cultural assimilation and kept connections with their culture and country alive by performing and exchanging traditional practices. Attempts to make a Catholic mission of the leprosarium were never entirely successful due to Protestant competition as well as the assertion by patients of their own religious choices.

C. Robson, *Missionary Women, Leprosy and Indigenous Australians, 1936–1986*, https://doi.org/10.1007/978-3-031-05796-0_6

The Work Ethic

Across the three institutions, and throughout their periods of operation, able-bodied patients, apart from young children, were expected to fulfil various tasks contributing to the day-to-day running of the leprosaria. Support by the staff and higher levels of administration for this practice did not stem from any single strand of thinking; rather, it represented a confluence of widely held and long ingrained societal values, current psycho-medical theory, and practical, fiscal considerations. Applied to Indigenous patients, and to various degrees, it was an imposition of Western morals and lifestyle; in its extreme, in the allocation of tedious or physically arduous tasks for little or no pay, it replicated a pattern of exploitation typified in European-Indigenous labour relations.

Work by patients was vital to the day-to-day maintenance of the institutions and for their own sustenance, health care, and other services. In the 1930s and 1940s when shortages of food, clothing, and other necessities were acute, patient labour forces were quickly formed, and equipped with lessons in thrift. To feed the patients after her arrival, Mother Peter at Fantome Island taught the female patients to bake bread and at Derby, they were shown how to sew flour bags into dresses for the girls.[1] The men were directed to chopping wood and helping with construction and transport. As time went on, and resources became more readily available, patient industry became more productive and organised, continuing to be distributed along lines of gender, physical ability, and proficiency. Women patients made and washed patients' clothes, milked animals, and fed the poultry while the men slaughtered stock, transported supplies, and operated motors for pumps and other equipment. Patients of both sexes assisted with nursing and showering the less mobile patients and cooking.[2] Those who came from missions or Europeanised backgrounds were given greater responsibility and delegated the less mundane tasks. Former nursing staff have emphasised the importance of the patients' roles as workers, stating that they were indispensable to the overall functioning of the institutions.[3]

The payment of wages to working patients varied over time, place, and their race. Those classified as "Aboriginal" were either not paid at all or very little. Indigenous patients worked as lumberjacks on Channel Island for no pay for several years prior to the 1950s, as did any patient working on Fantome Island for less than four hours.[4] By 1951, Indigenous patients at these places working full time were paid ten shillings a week. This compares with the forty shillings paid to workers on Indigenous government settlements.[5] Mixed descent patients employed in more authoritative or skilled work received two pound and ten at Channel Island in this period. On the basis that workers from outside the leprosarium demanded double pay rates to work at these institutions, officials calculated that the sixty-seven patients employed at Channel Island in 1953 saved the Commonwealth government £78,900 per year.[6]

As at government settlements, Indigenous patients only received a proportion of the wages. The balance was held in bank accounts and small amounts could be withdrawn with the permission of senior staff.[7] It is unclear whether this policy had always been in place or if it was introduced after paternalistic concerns were raised about the ability of Indigenous patients to use their money wisely. An article in the journal, *The Annals of Our Lady of the Sacred Heart* in 1952, conveyed the attitude of staff: "Brother gives them jobs and receives some money from the government to pay them…The stronger ones thus earn considerable sums at times but alas! They gamble the money away among themselves and send to Darwin for all sorts of food and costly articles" (Fig. 6.1).[8]

Work, as a form of mental and physical occupation, was also considered an essential part of leprosy treatment from at least the 1930s. In their authoritative textbook, copies of which were found on shelves in all Australian leprosaria, leprologists Leonard Rogers and Ernest Muir stated that work routines should be encouraged as physiotherapy:

> Work in the garden and in the field is excellent, and many of the deformities which render this impossible to the poorer patients would never have occurred if they had persisted in doing such work from the beginning.[9]

They also believed that work was "effective in preventing the dissemination of infection [and] extremely beneficial to the patient both mentally and physically."[10] The psychological problems associated with institutionalising leprosy sufferers were familiar to leprologists internationally:

> Left to himself, the condition of the leprous patient is a most deplorable one. The long duration of the disease, exclusion from work and from intercourse with his fellows, and the ostracism to which he is subjected cause mental depression, and sometimes even acute melancholia. Where lepers live in agricultural settlements, employment suited to their capacity

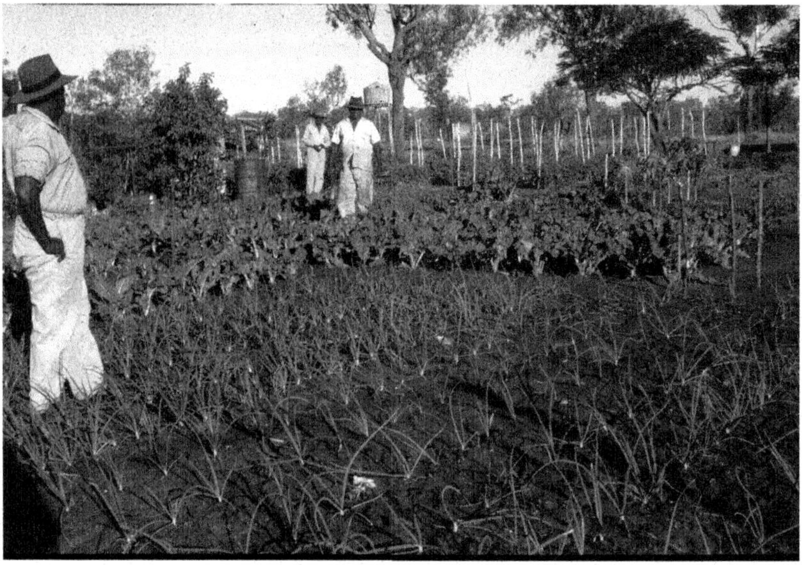

Fig. 6.1 Male patients working in vegetable garden, n.d., Derby Leprosarium (SSJG Heritage Centre Broome)

> for work and association with others who are in the same condition has a cheering effect upon them.[11]

Australian medico-bureaucrats agreed with this theory and endorsed its application in leprosaria under their control. In 1934, leprosy expert and Queensland health official, Raphael Cilento, advised the Commonwealth Director-General of Health, J.H.L. Cumpston, that leprosy patients should be given "purposive employment…in profitable farm work."[12] Western Australian Commissioner of Public Health, Everitt Atkinson, also supported these principles in planning the Derby leprosarium, adding a specification for recreational activity: "It is important that facilities for play and occupation are available…Everything must be done to divert the patient's mind from his unfortunate plight…".[13]

The view, as purported by Rogers and Muir above, that "exclusion from work" could cause depression, and that its resumption, even if repetitive and arduous, could lift a patient's spirits can be linked with the prevailing and more widely applied Australian work ethic. Hard work as morally edifying and a boost to one's sense of self-worth had permeated British social values since the eighteenth century. In colonial Australia, this idea was central to the reforming ideology of institutions such as asylums and charitable institutions.[14] Historian David Potts has argued for its persistence during the Great Depression when Australian men, unable to secure employment, felt the sting of their childhood adage, "Tis the idle grow weary…There's joy in labour found."[15] Without work, fears arose of dependency on others for assistance and the descent into pauperism, a state associated with "moral and spiritual inferiority."[16]

The 'rhetoric of pauperism' was frequently sounded by missionaries and administrators regarding Indigenous people, from the nineteenth century.[17] Mission leaders eschewed idleness and dependency in favour of creating "productive members of European society." In the interwar period, Indigenous affairs officials believed that the policy of social assimilation was contingent upon eliminating pauperism, Tim Rowse has argued. Protector of Aboriginals, J.W. Bleakley, declared, "Any system that pauperises the native, or produces for him without effort on his own part, is not likely to succeed in uplifting him."[18] F.E.A. Bateman, who led an official inquiry into Indigenous affairs in Western Australia saw Indigenous idleness as morally threatening to society, claiming, "the saying that the devil finds work for idle hands is particularly true when applied to the native."[19] Idleness became a fault to be corrected in the mission, the reserve, the institution—where so many Indigenous people were transferred from the late nineteenth to mid-twentieth centuries. And the performance of labour with little or no monetary compensation was the remedy.

The views of Catholic religious staff closely accorded with the official line. In writings to their religious superiors, they reported success in mobilising patients into work schedules. In 1940, Mother Peter, in her new role as leprosarium matron, lamented the inactivity of the patients, as her first journal entry reveals: "The condition of our poor people was in a very poor state. … At one end the people were quite idle and everything was very dirty." She made the allocation of jobs for them one of her first priorities:

> The first two weeks passed in trying to form plans, and in meeting and learning to know the people, and deciding what work or duty they could perform. Following on this, various duties were given the men, women, and children. They responded very well, thank God.[20]

On Channel Island, Brother McCarthy, the superintendent, organised work tasks among the patients, noting that "Some of the blacks are well able to chop wood and pump water" and that "some of the half-castes are good cooks and take turns about cooking for the other patients."[21] Similarly, in Derby, such industry was extolled, with one patient's hard work and achievements cause for the medical officer to recommend regular wage payments to him.[22]

The support by the religious staff of the leprosarium work ethic aligns with a Catholic tradition that values work as virtuous and indolence as vice. Michel Foucault has explored work as the central reforming strategy of the early modern institution of therapeutic confinement, arguing that both Catholic and Protestant authorities subscribed to this philosophy.[23] More familiar to leprosarium staff was the concurrent religious discourse. In 1931, Pope Pius XI expressed, first, the centrality of work to life: "man is born to labor as the bird to fly," and, second, its physical and spiritual virtue: "bodily labor, which Divine Providence decreed to be performed, even after original sin, for the good at once of man's body and soul…"[24] The virtue of manual labour and the demoralising nature of idleness were also emphasised in constitutions of the Catholic religious orders who, in their roles as teachers and priests, helped to define contemporary Catholic values.[25]

It is important not to overstate the dominance of labour in a patient's day. Most patients did not work for the whole day and certain hours were kept free for other activities discussed further. Patients had time off to go fishing or take up other leisurely activities, and the Sisters regularly packed up the truck and took them on excursions either for fishing or bush picnics. Each weekend, as related by one Sister, Channel Island patients were "free to take their rations and camp out. All look forward to these little outings and spend the time fishing, swimming etc. But there are always a few who are not well enough to go, and these are always cared for at home or taken by the others" (Fig. 6.2).[26]

School

With the admission of patients as young as seven, the Sisters at all three institutions established schools shortly after they assumed nursing duties.[27] Unlike the work policy, the schools were their own initiative. Government departments did not determine the curricula or provide educational materials or facilities until many years after the schools'

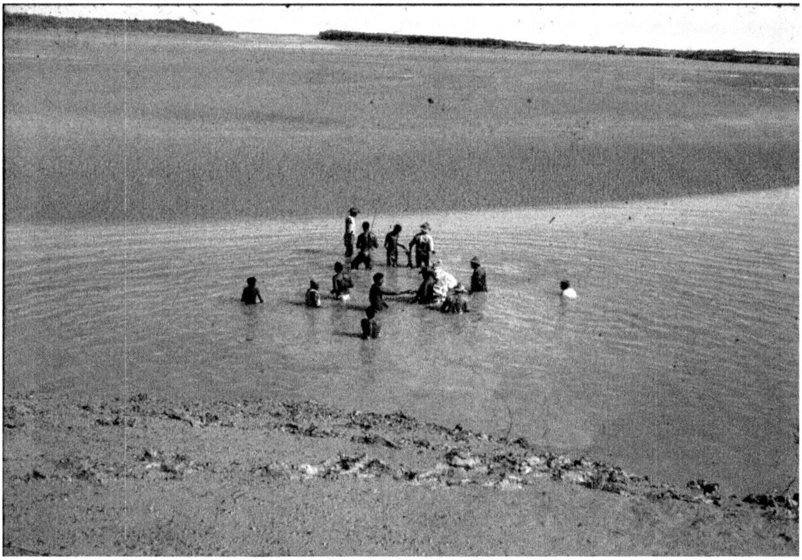

Fig. 6.2 Male patients from Derby Leprosarium on fishing trip, 1964–1969 (SSJG Heritage Centre Broome)

commencement. As with the work regimen, school classes introduced discipline to the patients and filled their time with wholesome occupation. They were also vehicles for furthering the Sisters' goals of assimilation and evangelisation. Classes were at first held in open gunyahs with dirt floors. Equipment and furniture consisted of what was donated or could be found in nature and adapted to use, such as blackboards and seating. Matrons doubled as schoolteachers, sometimes with the assistance of the more educated patients. Gradually, schoolteachers were recruited from the respective religious congregations, and classrooms were built and fitted out (Fig. 6.3).

Indigenous children were instructed in skills and moral values considered by the Sisters to be useful in the leprosarium and conducive to their 'civilising' and Christianising project. The lessons included English literacy, basic arithmetic, geography, hygiene, and religious education. Adult classes in literacy and numeracy were also offered. Literacy was of immediate use to the patients since it enabled them to write to family

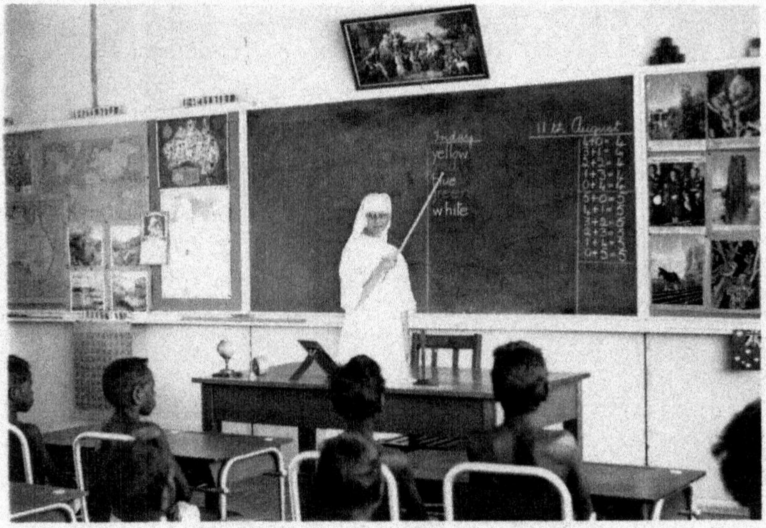

Fig. 6.3 Sr Mary Vincent Dayball teaching school at East Arm Leprosarium, 1950s (DOLSH Archives, Kensington, New South Wales)

members at home.[28] It was also core to the Western Christian education promoted by the Sisters and gave access to fundamental texts such as the Catholic catechism and Australian primary school readers. The Sisters' attempts to implant the Australian Catholic primary school in the leprosarium can be seen in a photograph of the classroom in the 1950s. Apart from the full class of Indigenous pupils, the room could have been in any such school. The dominant portrayal of western Christian civilisation apparent in the images of the British queen and Christ, and maps defining the triumphs of Western colonialisation, created what historian Christine Trimingham Jack has called a "symbolic landscape of our lives" and were "carriers of powerful messages about the right way of living."[29]

The leprosarium schools paid special attention to health and hygiene. Fantome Island schoolchildren were awarded prizes for consistently attending clinic for the painful injections of chaulmoogra oil and taught the consequences of poor hygiene through moral stories.[30] Cleanliness and tidiness were emphasised in the classroom, but not without the understanding that they were not easily achieved by children affected by leprosy. Mother Peter noted of her students in 1942, "Their little hands are mostly deformed or broken with bad blisters. It is difficult for them to keep their work in good order."[31] At Derby, the job of leprosarium schoolteacher, Sister Therese, was "to see that the classroom is attractive and clean, also that in the class room the pupils wear clean, neat clothes, that their hands are clean, their hair tidy."[32] Hygiene was obviously important in the leprosarium but its inextricable pairing with habits of tidiness as time-honoured practices drilled into the minds of Western school children indicate that it was encouraged as part of the overall 'civilising project,' rather than solely for sanitary purposes.

The conventional methods of reward and punishment applied also to leprosarium schoolchildren. As with prizes for complying with odious medical treatment, misbehaviour was dealt with by writing out lines. One young Derby patient, whose first experience of school was in the leprosarium, was once asked to mind the class: "So he got them singing and the kids started to laugh while they were singing, so he gave them a piece of paper each and made them write, 'I must not laugh while singing.'"[33] Another patient, who recounted his memories in song-form, remembered corporal punishment:

> Oh, it was real good living at Bungarun.
>
> You know, good friends,school
> We used to get a hiding too!
> We tried to run away from school.[34]

Evidence suggests that education beyond primary level was not offered in the leprosaria until the 1960s when it was combined with government correspondence school programmes. But even this basic education exceeded what was available to many Indigenous children generally.[35] Some ex-patients and their communities have seen the education acquired at the leprosarium school as an asset. Philomena Kerinaiua's only experience of school was at Channel Island, and the parents of a boy at Derby leprosarium "appreciated the good education he was receiving from the St John of God Sisters."[36] Bob Nyalcas of Turkey Creek thought that an education at the Derby leprosarium gave some people in his community an edge over others: "They bin do em good. When they bin young, yeh, they used to do em school there...they're really top class now."[37] In contrast, some people, from backgrounds with greater educational opportunities, were disadvantaged by the leprosarium school system. "John," a Fantome Island patient, recalled that school classes in the mid- to late 1940s only ran for two hours a day and that he "couldn't read or write much at all when [he] came out."[38] Meanwhile, his siblings had acquired qualifications in different trades and professions.

The Sisters' school classes were not the sole source of education for the leprosarium children. Contact with older patients from culturally diverse backgrounds led to their familiarisation with belief systems, customs and languages that varied widely from those promoted in the school. For example, patients learnt English in school, but they also sometimes continued to speak their own languages and, through meeting patients from other language groups, became adept multi-lingual speakers. Philomena Kerinaiua explained,

> I lost count of my own language. I guess you could say I never spoke my own language since when I left from here and I go to that quarantine. We used to just talk Kriol or English. Then they took me to the Tiwi Islands and I learned little bit of language there, Tiwi language.[39]

Another patient learnt "English, Kuninjku, Tiwi Lingo, Oenpelli languages and Mawu" while in the leprosarium but lost the use of her native language.[40]

One former nursing Sister stated that during her time from the late 1940s to the 1960s, staff did not attempt to prevent patients speaking in their own language, although conceded that this was not the case in the missions.[41] The staff tolerated a range of practices that varied from the Western Christian model they actively promoted, as will be demonstrated further in this chapter. Even had they wanted to suppress them, they did not have the ultimate authority to do so in a government institution, but, more likely they recognised the benefits of patients maintaining certain aspects of their culture.

Music, Art, and Dance

Organised music activities were an important element of institutional life and included instrumental and singing instruction, bands and ensembles, and concert performances. Music tuition in schools and privately by Catholic Sisters has a strong tradition in Australia and they played a significant role in the popularisation of piano lessons in the early twentieth century. Teaching European music in the leprosarium imparted this cultural tradition to the Indigenous patients.[42] The Sisters used music also as therapy, to distract the patients from the distress of their circumstances and to circumvent their own methods of amelioration which, in some cases, threatened the safety of the institution. The playing of musical instruments by the patients satisfied yet one more objective of the Sisters, at least in the case of the Derby leprosarium: it was a form of physiotherapy.

The most formal and comprehensive music programme occurred at Derby, initiated by Mother Alphonsus Daly, who, in addition to her nursing qualifications, was a trained musician. In the 1940s, she began teaching violin to five patients for a music ensemble, which gradually developed into an orchestra of forty violins, six banjos, a cello, a cornet, and several percussion instruments. Performances were given to official visitors to the leprosarium. In addition, patients were taught singing, drama, and dance, and participated in concerts held in the operating theatre. At the island institutions, the Sisters encouraged music and song, and taught hymns and carols, formed patient bands, and organised concerts.[43]

The Derby patients learnt to play their instruments "by ear". Rather than learning to read music, they listened to Mother Alphonsus play the piano and imitated the melodies on their different instruments. Students who developed greater competence were placed in the front rows, with the others following their lead.[44] Having taught music in Broome for many years, Mother Alphonsus attributed the success of this system to her belief that "Aborigines are a naturally musical people with a keen sense of harmony, melody and rhythm" and a "love and memory for music."[45] Her successor after 1964, Sydney Conservatorium-trained Sister Camille continued this method and thought that, compared with the European students whom she had taught, "Aborigines had a gift... they'd hear a new tune and would catch on...the patients continued to learn this way after radios and tape recorders became available" (Fig. 6.4).[46]

At Mother Alphonsus' request, the health department initially provided the musical instruments and funded their repair and string replacements, a constant requirement due to the high humidity.[47] More instruments were made available after the Catholic periodical, *The Advocate*, asked readers to donate them as an act of charity "to these poor unfortunates."[48] Mother Alphonsus held music practice sessions at least

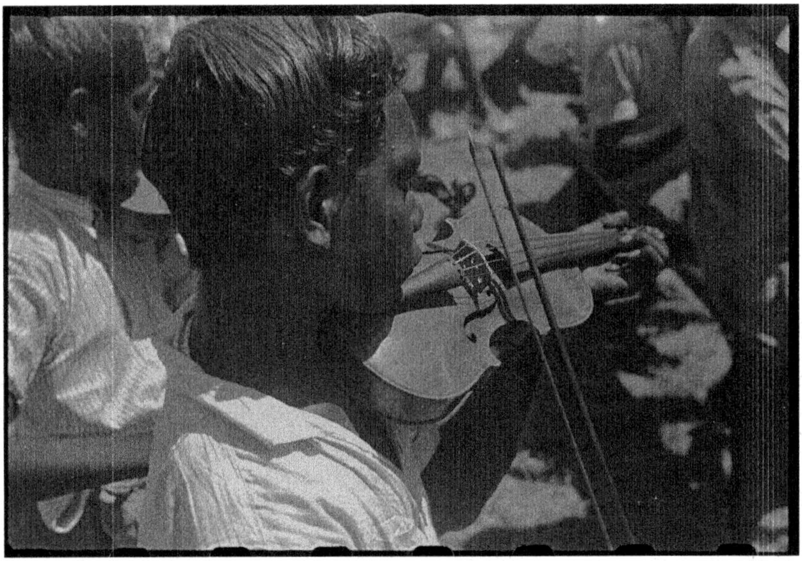

Fig. 6.4 Violinist, Derby Leprosarium Orchestra 1948 (Stuart Gore Collection, State Library of Western Australia)

three evenings a week, ran a patient choir and gave dancing lessons. By the 1950s, she had added jazz and honky tonk to the orchestra's classical repertoire and "we'd play *Danny Boy* and *Down by the Swanee* and sing away like nobody's business."[49] Considerable effort went to the design and making of outfits such as cowboy suits for the boys and white dresses for the girls for the many concerts held. One former patient recalled Mother Alphonsus' fastidious attention: "Oh she wanted everything proper, you know Mother. Big bosses would come from Perth whenever Aboriginal people did concerts. We would have a big night."[50]

Music lessons and concerts were another means of inculcating the patients with Western culture, and more specifically, that typifying early to mid-twentieth century Catholic schools. Along with the technical skills, patients were taught the conventions of dress and etiquette, the discipline of regular practice and the appreciation of European music from various genres and historical periods. For Catholic religious Sisters, training children, particularly girls, in the performing arts was considered *de rigueur*, and essential to their cultural refinement.[51] At girls' schools, proficiency in piano-playing was prized as a marker of female gentility, and at Catholic boys' schools, Jesuit Brothers introduced music and drama lessons to counter the rough and tumble of sports activities.[52] Educators saw lessons in the performing arts as a civilising process.

The leprosarium Sisters considered music, dance, and theatre to be therapeutic for the patients. Mother Alphonsus coined the phrase 'The Therapy of Distraction' to describe the immersion of patients in these activities, which she considered enjoyable and diverting, to stave off boredom and melancholia.[53] Sister Camille stated that music was "compensation for long periods without family and land."[54] Former patients remembered that music "was an escape from confinement" and that it "was to keep us occupied instead of thinking about our relations."[55] Their testimonies confirm the perception of a journalist who visited Derby in 1949 and was treated to a concert given by the orchestra: "...the rapt expression of their faces as violins, cellos, and drums followed the notes of the piano showed the enthusiasm with which they entered into this form of relaxation."[56]

Music was also used to steer the patients away from activities considered harmful or morally undesirable, such as sexual liaisons, drinking alcohol and gambling. Former nursing Sisters remember the orchestra as Mother Alphonsus' way of keeping the men away from the women. Sister Angela recalled "sometimes a number of them would be missing from practice - struck by the gambling fever... I used to go around the camps and persuade them to go to practice."[57] That music was seen as a possible substitute for the gratification derived from these pastimes is telling of the importance it held for the Sisters themselves. Music could be empowering, especially to those whose sensuality and other forms of personal expression was by necessity subdued, as Australian Catholic schoolgirls and the Sisters who had taught them had long recognised.[58] Mother Alphonsus, who from a young age was a woman of "great stories, comic songs, grand opera" found joy in musical achievement.[59] At Fantome Island, too, the Sisters' own enjoyment of music, and their enthusiasm in drawing the patients to its appeal, has been often recalled. These women were, then, exemplars as well as instructors, of the moral and spiritual value of music, song, and dance in their own lives. And while this strategy targeted the patients' personal well-being, it also helped to further the institutions' public health goals of maintaining sexual segregation and law and order.

The 'Therapy of Distraction' helped patients to cope with a situation that they were unable to change, the underlying principle being the same as that for "play and occupation," as originally recommended by medical officers. Music potentially offered more personal satisfaction than menial work or simple hobbies. As one patient put it, "I always looked forward to practice time because it was something different, and you had your mind set on learning…It helped lift spirits up just like a real orchestra band."[60] Mother Alphonsus' use of a structured music programme to address the patients' psychosocial needs is reminiscent of distraction techniques used more recently in clinical psychiatry, which advocate that patients "maximize engagement in activities …provid[ing] a sense of pleasure and mastery."[61]

Mother Alphonsus also promoted the playing of music as physiotherapy. Stringed instruments such as the violin, cello, banjo, and guitar require the use of fine and sometimes complex motor skills by the fingers. Wind instruments, too, such as the cornet, were taught, requiring the regular pumping of the valves by the fingers to produce notes of different pitch. The patients were told that instrument-playing was encouraged in order "to get the fingers moving."[62]

The limbs most commonly subjected to disability in leprosy are the hands.[63] According to one guide on leprosy care published in 1968, "every patient should ensure that every joint of every paralysed finger should be passed passively throughout its whole range of movement at least once a day [since] a badly contracted hand is forever the silent witness of neglect."[64] Playing stringed instruments does not exactly replicate these movements but the required flexibility ensures considerable and regular exercising of the finger joints. In the absence of a funded professional physiotherapy programme, the incorporation of music was an important improvisation: it was self-monitoring (as if the fingers were not stretched enough, the desired sound would not be produced) and it took no more time or persuasion than the practice of music itself.

Despite the Sisters' enthusiasm for European creative arts, they were tolerant, and, indeed, supportive of traditional dance and song performed by the patients.[65] Fantome Island Sisters regularly attended corroborees and other dancing performed each Saturday night at the invitation of the patients from the early 1940s.[66] At Derby, it was similar. Sister Dunne remembered that "When darkness fell, the sound of the old men singing, the clapping of sticks and the didgeridoo could be heard. When there were enough men and women well enough to dance, they would have corroborees."[67] When visitors came to Fantome Island in the late 1950s, the patients would "perform lively corroborees, the natives decorating and painting themselves with clay and cockatoo feathers, also they entertain with Island songs and musical instruments, blowing through gum leaves..." (Fig. 6.5).[68]

According to one former music teacher at Derby, corroborees served the same purpose as the Derby orchestra: they were encouraged because "music was so important to the people."[69] They were the alternative for patients who were unable or unwilling to swap tradition for European ways, often due to their advancing age. The Sisters' approval of corroborees reflected the concurrent Australian Catholic missiology which supported traditional practices if they did not violate Christian principles.[70] Pope Pius XII's 1951 mission encyclical, *Evangelii Praecones*, stated, "...let not the Gospel on being introduced into any new land destroy or extinguish whatever its people possess that is naturally good, just or beautiful."[71] "Bush corroborees" consisting mainly of dance,

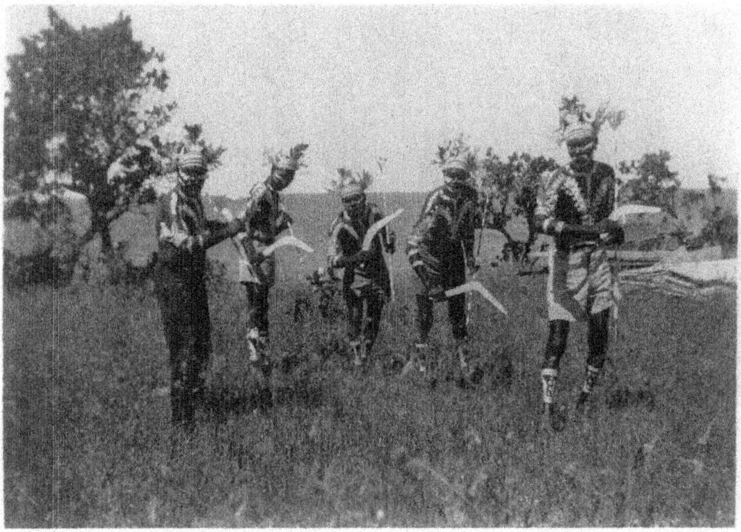

Fig. 6.5 Indigenous dancers at Fantome Island Leprosarium (James Cook University Library Special Collections)

costume and song were acceptable to Catholic missionaries, but not male initiation rituals and "bone-pointing corroborees" (Fig. 6.6).[72]

Artwork and handcrafts flourished at all leprosaria. Painting and sculpting were encouraged for their therapeutic properties but also, through the styles and motifs employed, were ways for patients to keep the memories and connections with their homes alive. At Derby, from at least 1945, some patients took up the local tradition of engraving and painting boab nuts.[73] Ngarinyin man and noted boab carver, Francis Dolby, explained on a video how creating this artform was "relaxing" and it "gets your mind off everything."[74] The carved images reference Indigenous creation stories and feature the Wandjina spirit or animals such as turtles and owls. Dolby's comments that this artform "connects you to Wandjina and the country" and that the finished product makes him "feel kinder strong…and proud" help to clarify its importance for leprosarium patients, forced away from their lands and people.[75] In adult education classes, patients also made and designed mats, wall hangings and

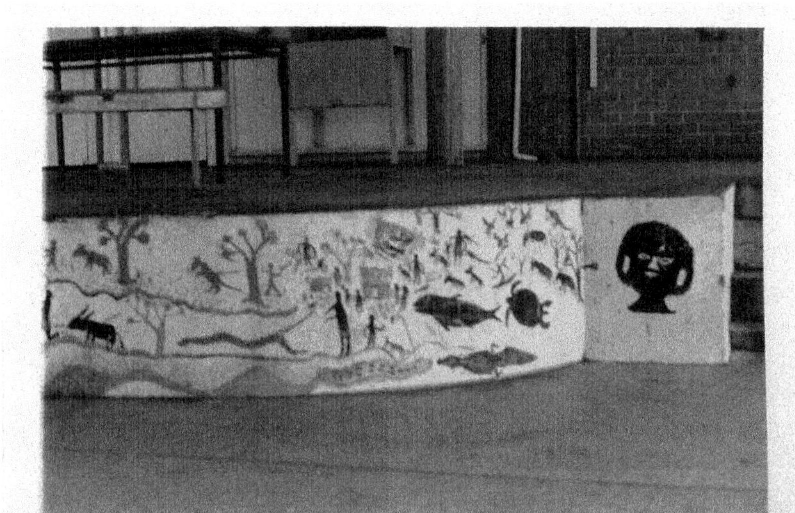

Fig. 6.6 Patients' artwork, Channel Island recreation hall (DOLSH Archives, Kensington, New South Wales)

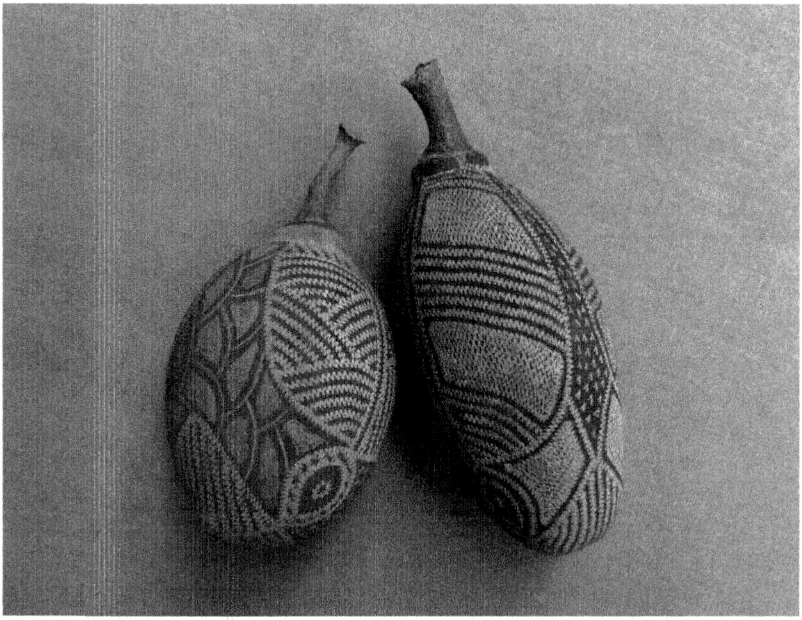

Fig. 6.7 Carved boab nuts by Adriel Archie (Photo by Amelia Robson. Author's collection)

wood sculptures, and entered them into competitions at local art festivals.[76] Leprosarium patients from about the 1960s sold their paintings and handcrafts to the public. One former Derby patient, Waddi Boyoi, recalls selling the boomerangs he made so that he could give money to his young son. He implied that this was a way of fulfilling his paternal role which had been disrupted when he entered the leprosarium (Fig. 6.7).[77]

Christianity

As missionaries, the Sisters saw the patients' faith and spiritual welfare as integral to their stewardship at the leprosaria. It was important to introduce Catholicism to the Protestants and non-Christians and to help the Catholics maintain and strengthen their faith for the difficult path ahead. But, while evangelisation was expected on a mission station, its place in a leprosarium, a government secular institution, was questionable, especially to missionaries of other denominations. Sectarian division and official scrutiny led some Sisters to temper their evangelistic efforts. Some senior administrators, however, did not object to making Christians, or even Catholics of the patients, and perhaps hadn't expected the Sisters to leave their mission mandates behind when appointed. Yet some Catholic male clergy, determined to implant the Church within these institutions, thought the Sisters didn't try hard enough to evangelise the patients. The Sisters, therefore, had to negotiate the multiple and sometimes contradictory expectations of their spiritual and worldly masters. Many patients nonetheless converted to Catholicism while others retained their existing beliefs or adopted the faith of competing Protestants.

The Sisters' primary concern, however, was the maintenance of their own religious practices, including access to religious services. Rooms at the convents served as their private chapels and local priests were assigned to visiting the institutions for their Mass and confession. Catholic patients made up only a small minority at each leprosarium when the Sisters first arrived and, except at Fantome Island, Catholic religious practices were kept understated and mostly took place within the Sisters' precincts, set well away from the patient accommodation and other common facilities. Although the priests and chapels were intended for the Sisters and Catholic patients, they became crucial to patient proselytisation, as will be discussed.

On Fantome Island, the missionary impulse was energetically pursued. Soon after the leprosarium opened, Mother Peter gave daily religious instruction and prayer meetings for the patients. She recorded the presence of five Catholic patients initially but documented the attendance of five "aspirants."[78] She kept count of Catholic patients, noting baptisms and attendances at prayer meetings, masses, and religious instruction.[79] "Come the day, when they all will be Catholics, but it is not yet," she told the bishop of Townsville, Hugh Ryan, two years after her arrival.[80]

Mother Peter was leprosarium Superior between 1940 and 1945 when the patient death toll was at its highest, and she baptised every patient she could before they gave their last breath. Of the fourteen deaths in 1940, at least ten were baptised into the Catholic Church shortly before their deaths, using the provision *periculo mortis* (in danger of death), or, less often, in *articulo mortis* (at the point of death).[81] For prospective converts to the Catholic faith, including former Presbyterians, Anglicans and Baptists, baptisms were conducted *sub conditione*, allowing for "doubts as to the validity of their former Baptism."[82] As these patients were dying, we cannot be certain of their consent, but at least one, a fourteen-year-old girl, resisted just hours before her death. When a Sister began the baptismal rites, she "was told off in no uncertain or lady like terms."[83] A patient who was leader of the leprosarium Baptist community agreed to administer the baptism under the Sister's instructions, and the girl reportedly acquiesced and died peacefully.[84]

The Fantome Island Sisters were mostly left unhindered to pursue their missionary ends with the patients, largely because government officials spared neither the time nor interest to intervene. Superintendent Julian, for the time he was present, was an active Catholic and ally to the Sisters until his departure in 1947 after which the Palm Island superintendent took the role at a distance. Senior administrators, such as Cilento, Hanlon, and Bleakley, also supported the Sisters, grateful for their taking on the "repulsive" leprosarium work.[85] The only person monitoring their religious activities was the elderly Anglican chaplain of Palm Island, Ernest Gribble, who, until the late 1940s, made the rocky boat ride across to Fantome Island once a week to minister to his flock of patients, ever diminishing due to the growing menace of "the Romans".[86] Few heeded his complaints. After his retirement, Catholicism eventually superseded the Church of England as the dominant religion, in part owing to the installation of a resident Catholic priest. One former patient recalls his schoolmates gradually being converted Catholicism while he remained one of the few Anglicans. He does not recall any overt approaches by the Sisters to join their faith, just their suggestions to the very ill that they should be prepared for death, and his attraction to the Catholic hymns.[87]

At Derby, the Sisters were not as free to practise and spread their faith. The appointment of a resident lay superintendent with authority over the Sisters enabled greater surveillance and checks on their activities. Wyburt Powell, appointed in 1937, was the first of several superintendents to regularly report on the Sisters' conduct to their superiors. His complaints about the priest who came to say Mass for the Sisters and Catholic patients were seen by medical officer, Albert Davis, as arising from

> a difference of religion. Powell is a matter of fact man who does not take kindly to the priest periodically parading the leprosarium in the robes of his office and claims that the Beagle Bay inmates receive favouritism over their unconverted brothers.[88]

In response, the Under-Secretary, Frederick Huelin, reminded the Sisters that

> the leprosarium is a government institution ... We have no objection whatever to any of the patients who desire the assistance and consolation of your religion receiving it, but anything...that might be interpreted as a general observance or ceremony, or open public demonstration of religious practices will only cause embarrassment to the Department and yourselves.[89]

Huelin was clearly not worried about the Sisters' practising their faith or even evangelising the patients; he was concerned about the visibility of these actions, giving the impression of a government-funded Catholic institution. In an era of intense sectarian rivalry, a Protestant public would not be impressed. Powell's objections may well have been in defence of the patients, but as a supporter of the United Aborigines Mission (UAM), a Protestant body, sectarian hostility may also have been the motive. Following Powell's death in 1939, a succession of superintendents connected with the UAM and the Presbyterian missions was appointed. Whether the policy was deliberate to keep Catholic dominance in check or reflected a preponderance of men of these denominations in the Kimberley cannot be ascertained. In the battle for Indigenous souls, accusations flew in both directions. The Catholic priest complained that the superintendent deliberately stranded him at the airport to prevent his leprosarium visitation while superintendents petitioned the government to cease the practice of transferring leprosarium newborns to Catholic missions.[90]

Regardless of such monitoring, a small pamphlet from the Sisters of John of God in 1954 claimed that "numbers of converts have been made within the last ten years amongst the pagan lepers and now there is a huge Catholic community."[91] The Sisters communicated their beliefs in less obvious ways, for example, through school lessons and evening rosary recitals which took the form of Mother Gertrude's social gatherings.[92] An important conduit for transmitting the Catholic faith, without the presence of the Sisters, were the patient catechists. Gregory Howard, originally from Beagle Bay Mission, and Theresa Puertollano, a former Catholic convent student, were designated catechists from the early 1940s and took charge of the rosaries and school classes for the boys and girls, respectively.[93] Ex-patient and former Beagle Bay Mission resident, Eileen Pan, described how Catholicism spread to people from the Kimberley cattle stations:

> But one thing we never forgot was our rosary. Every evening, five o'clock we'd all get together and say our rosary and of course people from the station used to come and ask us,
>
> > "What you people say?"
> > "We saying our rosary to Our Lady."
> > "What about you teach'em us too?"
>
> So, one day, Theresa Puertollano started them off with the rosary. It was all the little stations that now are so big, pastoral stations. They used to come and we'd all say rosary.[94]

Puertollano herself remembered:

> I was the one that used to take all the people for catechism in my spare time. Every evening when I had nothing to do, I'd call the ladies, they used to come and I'd make them sit down. Most of them came from Turkey Creek, Wyndham, places like that.[95]

As well as taking rosary and religious instruction, she sang hymns with the Catholic patients, and seemed to have attracted others to do the same:

> We had lovely lawns there and ladies would come and sit, and men, some of the men to sing hymns from the footpaths, they would join in with us, and I'd have the little kids in front. We'd always sing a hymn. Hail Queen of Heaven was the first, the favourite.[96]

Biblical stories and messages imparted by mission people of mixed descent who shared circumstances as leprosarium patients and racial and cultural origins with the Indigenous people they taught, were more likely to have a greater impact than if coming from European religious. They were delivered in a non-coercive benign manner in a social atmosphere. Christianity was far more palatable introduced this way, compared with direct approaches by white missionaries whose motives were tainted with the depredatory deeds of their compatriots.

On Channel Island, young Indigenous patients from the Catholic missions on the Tiwi Islands also possibly drew converts to the Church. They were not formal catechists but set examples as devout Catholics, as noted by Fr William Henschke: "They are such good Catholics and go to Mass and Benediction on Sundays and may help win others to the faith."[97] He considered that the prospect of further Tiwi admissions would "swell our Catholics on Channel Island."[98]

Henschke was disappointed with the first leprosarium Sisters for not actively trying to evangelise the patients. His letter to his Provincial Superior praised their nursing work but he complained,

> they are nurses only…I thought the Sisters would have a big influence on the patients and turn them to the faith. …They don't mix with the patients or even invite them up to the convent…if the Sisters showed an interest in them they would gradually win them over and if they had sacraments and prayer to help them, they would have a chance of bettering their lives.[99]

This criticism may reflect more on the massive workload of the first Channel Island Sisters, as described in their communications back to their Sydney motherhouse.[100] Or it might also reveal the variability with which missionaries carried out their individual vocations, highlighting the act of nursing as a Christian apostolate, without the need for other interventions. As one priest wrote of Sister nurses, "To save souls [they] occupy themselves first of all, with the bodies of the natives… [The Sister] brings to them also the comfort of her smile, to bring hope or resignation."[101] But this was not enough for the zealous Henschke, who had waited so long and pushed so hard to have a Catholic leprosarium. He soon had one of the Sisters replaced with "a capable person [who] has a great personality."[102] This anecdote shows that fulfilment of roles both as nurse for the government and missionary for the Church placed some Sisters in a difficult and sometimes impossible position, and the constraints on female missionary activity by the Catholic male hierarchy.

Notes

1. Anderson, Mother Peter to Ryan, Bishop Hugh, March 6, 1940 (1148, Box 57, Folder No. 924), Townsville Cathedral Archives (TCA).
2. Dunne, Sister Francis, 'Speech,' March 8, 2002 (2.21Y), Sisters of St John of God Archives Broome, Western Australia (SSJGB).

3. Whelan, Sister Marion OLSH. Interview with author. Typed transcript. Recorded at Kensington, New South Wales, August 12, 2008; Carroll, Sister Benedicta OLSH. Interview with author. Typed transcript. Recorded at Kensington, New South Wales, September 9, 2008.
4. Palm Island Superintendent to Deputy Director, Department of Native Affairs, September 1951 (Director of Native Affairs Office, 3A/153, Correspondence, Aboriginal and Torres Strait Islander, ITM505017), Queensland State Archives (QSA); Metcalfe, A.J. (Commonwealth Director-General of Health) to Watsford, Stephen (Northern Territory Director of Health, April 4, 1951 (A1658, 756/11/3, PART 1), National Archives of Australia (NAA).
5. Metcalfe to Secretary, Public Service Board, March 1, 1951 (A1658, 756/11/3, PART 1), NAA.
6. Acting Deputy Director, Northern Territory Department of Health to Metcalfe, April 17, 1953 (A1658, 756/11/3, PART 1), NAA.
7. 'List of Wages for the Fortnight Ending 21/6/1958' (Fantome Island) (Director of Native Affairs Office, Palm Island, GF/1, Correspondence, Aboriginal and Torres Strait Islander, ID ITM714734), QSA.
8. Morris, H.D. 1952. 'Darwin and Channel Island.' *The Annals of Our Lady of the Sacred Heart*, October 1, 229.
9. Rogers, Leonard and Ernest Muir. 1946. *Leprosy*, third edition. Baltimore: The Williams and Wilkins Co., 247.
10. Ibid., 248.
11. Ibid., 205–206.
12. Cilento, Raphael (Queensland Director-General of Health and Medical Services) to Cumpston, J.H.L., July 31, 1934 (A1928, 635/34), NAA.
13. Western Australia Public Health Department. 1936. *Report of the Public Health Department for the Year 1935–1936*. Perth: Department of Public Health, 8.
14. Garton, Stephen. 1990. *Out of Luck: Poor Australians and Social Welfare 1788–1988*. Sydney: Allen and Unwin, 54, 57, 59–61.
15. Potts, David. 2007. 'A Battle for the Mind: The Work Ethic during the Great Depression.' *Agora* 42 (4), 17.
16. O'Brien, Anne. 2011. 'Pauperism Revisited.' *Australian Historical Studies* 42 (2), 212.
17. Ibid., 212, 225–227.
18. J.W. Bleakley cited in Rowse, Tim. 1998. *White Flour, White Power: From Rations to Citizenship in Central Australia*. Cambridge and Melbourne: Cambridge University Press, 27.
19. Bateman, F.E.A. 1948. *Report on Survey of Native Affairs*. Perth: Government Printer, 11.
20. Our Lady Help of Christians (OLHC). Monthly Journal, Fantome Island, March 1940 (1144, Box 57, Folder 920), TCA.

21. McCarthy, Brother Dennis (Superintendent, Channel Island) to Kerrins, Fr Joseph (MSC Provincial Superior), September 28, 1943 (Provincial Correspondence, N.T. Darwin, 1943), Missionaries of the Sacred Heart Archives Kensington (MSCK).
22. Davis, Albert to Atkinson, Everitt, May 20, 1937 (PHD, 1935/0251, Cons 1003), State Records Office Western Australia (SROWA).
23. Foucault, Michel. 1967. *Madness and Civilization: A History of Insanity in the Age of Reason*. Trans. Richard Howard. London and New York: Routledge, 51.
24. Pope Pius XI 'Quadragesimo Anno.' *The Vatican*, http://www.vatican.va/holy_father/pius_xi/encyclicals/documents/hf_p-xi_enc_19310515_quadragesimo-anno_en.html (accessed 24 October 2009), sections 61 and 135.
25. Missionaries of the Sacred Heart. 1914. *Statutes for the Australian Province of the Missionaries of the Sacred Heart of Jesus*. Kensington: Missionaries of the Sacred Heart, No. 45, 9.
26. 'Channel Island' in *Smile of Mary,* (a newsletter of the Daughters of Our Lady of the Sacred Heart, Christimas 1943.
27. OLHC Monthly Journal, Fantome Island, June 1940 (1144, Box 57, Folder 920), TCA; 'Educational Involvement SSJG' (2.23F), SSJGB; Secretary, Department of Army to Secretary, Prime Minister's Department, November 1945 (A461, G347/1/10 PART 1), NAA.
28. Doolan, Sister Therese. Leprosarium School Report. n.d. (2.92B), SSJGB.
29. Trimingham Jack, Christine. 2003. *Growing Good Catholic Girls: Education and Convent Life in Australia*. Carlton: Melbourne University Press, 72.
30. "John" (former patient, Fantome Island Leprosarium). Interview with author. 7 June 2011. Typed transcript. Location and name confidential.
31. OLHC Monthly Journal, Fantome Island, July 1942 (1144, Box 57, Folder 920), TCA.
32. Doolan, Leprosarium School Report.
33. Wright, Edie. 2001. *Full Circle: From Mission to Community—A Family Story*. Fremantle: Fremantle Arts Centre Press, 211.
34. Michael Jambarra quoted in *Booroola Nganka (Derby Stories)*, ed. Colleen Hattersley, 2001, Derby: Yuriny Aboriginal Cultural Centre, 3; 'Bungarun' is the Indigenous name for Derby Leprosarium.
35. Regarding scarce education opportunities for Indigenous children in Western Australia, see Massam, Katherine. 2020. *A Bridge Between: Spanish Benedictine Missionary Women in Australia*. Canberra: Australian National University Press, 270.
36. Kerinaiua, Philomena. c. 2002. 'Philomena's Story.' In *So Far From Home: Oral Histories of the Stolen Generations*, ed. Lana Quall. Katherine:

Diwurruwurru-jaru Aboriginal Corporation, 28; Wright, *Full Circle*, 210.

37. Cited in Helen Ross. 1989. *Community Social Impact Assessment: A Cumulative Study in the Turkey Creek Area, Western Australia*, East Kimberley Working Paper, no. 27. Canberra: East Kimberley Impact Assessment Project, 47.
38. "John," Interview with author.
39. Kerinaiua, 'Philomena's Story,' 29. 'Quarantine' is a term some Indigenous people use to refer to Channel Island leprosarium as the site was originally a quarantine station.
40. Kildea, Sue. 2005. Birthing in the Bush: It's Time to Listen. Ph.D. Diss., University of Technology Sydney, 170.
41. Carroll, Sister Benedicta, Interview with author.
42. Griffiths, Paul. 2006. *New Penguin Dictionary of Music*. USA: Penguin Books, 247; Walsh, Margaret. 2001. *The Good Sams: Sisters of the Good Samaritan 1857–1969*. Mulgrave: John Garratt Publishing, 278.
43. Boyd, Sandy. 198–? Interview with Siobhan McHugh, Siobhan McHugh Collection of Australian Social History. Sound recording (ORAL TRC 2761/5), National Library of Australia; Chief Medical Officer to Metcalfe, November 15, 1950 (A1658, 756/11/3 PART 1), NAA.
44. Ex-patient in 'Healing Sounds of the Bungarun Orchestra,' *Message Stick*, DVD recording, Sydney: ABC Television, 1999.
45. Daly, Sister Alphonus M. 1986. *Healing Hands: Memories and Milestones of the Derby Leprosarium*. Perth: Health Department of Western Australia, 1986.
46. Poidevin, Sister Camille SJG. Interview with author. Typed transcript. Recorded at Derby, Western Australia, November 17, 2008.
47. Daly, *Healing Hands*.
48. Daly, G.C. 1947. 'Australia's Largest Leper Hospital.' *The Advocate*, April 23, 15.
49. Daly, *Healing Hands*; Gore, Stuart. 1951. *Walkabout*, November 1, 20; Ex-patient in *Healing Sounds of the Bungarun Orchestra*.
50. Puertollano, Theresa. 1997. 'These Were the Girls Who Left Broome for Beagle Bay.' In *The Telling of Stories: A Spiritual Journey of Kimberley Aboriginal People*, ed. Peter Bibby. Western Australia: Catholic Education Office, Kimberley Region, 51.
51. O'Brien, Anne. 2005. *God's Willing Workers: Women and Religion in Australia*. Sydney: University of New South Wales Press, 207–209; Walsh, *The Good Sams*, 336–337.
52. O'Brien, *God's Willing Workers*, 208; O'Donoghue, Tom and Stephanie Burley. 2008. 'God's Antipodean Teaching Force: An Historical Exposition on Catholic Teaching Religious in Australia.' *Teaching and Teacher Education* 24 185.

53. Daly, *Healing Hands*.
54. Sister Camille in *Healing Sounds of the Bungarun Orchestra*.
55. Former patient in *Healing Sounds of the Bungarun Orchestra*.
56. Ewers, J.K. 1949. 'Derby.' *Walkabout*, May 1, 39.
57. Moroney, Sister Angela. 'Reminiscences.' (2.1A), SSJGB.
58. O'Brien, Anne. 1995. 'Lifting the Lid.' *Eureka Street* 5 (6), 33.
59. Murnane, Sister Ignatius. n.d. 'A Chaplet of Dolours' (Papers of Joyce Caroline Dunphy, 6140A/45, MN 2305), Battye Library.
60. Former patient in *Healing Sounds of the Bungarun Orchestra*.
61. Clark, David M. 2009. 'Cognitive Behaviour Therapy for Anxiety Disorders.' In *New Oxford Textbook of Psychiatry*, ed. Michael G. Gelder, Nancy C. Andreasen, Juan J. López-Ibor Jr. and John R. Geddes, Oxford: Oxford University Press, 1285–1318; Osborne, Linda L., and Judith Fry McComish. 2006. 'Working with Borderline Personality Disorder: Nursing Interventions Using Dialectical Behavioral Therapy.' *Journal of Psychosocial Nursing & Mental Health Services* 44 (6), 40.
62. Former patient in *Healing Sounds of the Bungarun Orchestra;* Wright, *Full Circle*, 211.
63. Moschella, Samuel L. 2004. 'An Update on the Diagnosis and Treatment of Leprosy.' *Journal of the American Academy of Dermatology* 51 (3), 424.
64. Northern Territory Medical Service. 1986. *Leprosy in Northern Territory Aborigines: A Short Guide for Nursing Sisters in the Diagnosis, Treatment and Management of Leprosy in Aborigines*. Darwin: Northern Territory Medical Service, 24.
65. Former patient "A" (name withheld). Interview with Christine Choo, 1992, sound recording, State Library of Western Australia.
66. Mother Peter to Bishop Ryan, March 3, 1940 and April 7, 1941 (1148, Box 57, no.924), TCA.
67. Dunne, Sister Francis, Speech, March 8, 2002 (2.21Y), SSJGB.
68. Fantome Island Monthly Letters, Aug/Sept 1958, Franciscan Missionaries of Mary Archives, Summer Hill (FMMS).
69. Sister Camille, Interview with author.
70. Hearn, Peter. 2003. *A Theology of Mission: An Analysis of the Theology of Mission of the Catholic Diocese of Darwin in Its Ministry to Aboriginal People During the Episcopy of John O'Loughlin MSC 1949–85*. Kensington: Nelen Yubu Missiological Unit, 79–80.
71. Pope Pius XII. 1951. 'Evangelii Praecones' *The Vatican*. http://www.vatican.va/holy_father/pius_xii/encyclicals/documents/hf_p-xii_enc_02061951_evangelii-praecones_en.html (accessed 15 March 2010), Clause 56.
72. Hearn, *A Theology of Mission*, 37–38, 78–82.

73. Cardell-Oliver, F. 1945. 'The North-West: A Woman's Impression.' *The West Australian*, July 18, 7.
74. Dolby, Francis Xavier. 2016. 'The Boab Carver.' Video. Produced by Desert River Sea; Kimberley Art Then & Now, Art Gallery of Western Australia. Coordinated by Mowanjum Art & Culture Centre and Katie Breckon. https://vimeo.com/200112479. Accessed 2 February 2022.
75. Ibid.
76. Doolan Leprosarium School Report.
77. Boyoi, Waddi quoted in Shaw, Bruce. 1992. *When the Dust Come In Between: Aboriginal Viewpoints in the East Kimberley Prior to 1982.* Canberra: Aboriginal Studies Press, 140.
78. Mother Peter to Bishop Ryan, May 12, 1940 (1146, Box 57, Folder 924), TCA.
79. OLHC Monthly Journal, Fantome Island (1144, Box 57, Folder 920), TCA.
80. Mother Peter to Bishop Ryan, March 21, 1942 (1145, Box 57, Folder 921), TCA.
81. 'Fantome and Palm Islands Baptism Register,' TCA; 'Index of Patients' (Fantome Island Records D2), FMMS.
82. 'Converts: Rites to be Observed when Receiving Converts into the Church.' *Australasian Catholic Directory*. Sydney: Australasian Catholic Directory, 1941, 92.
83. Moloney, Fr. Patrick to Kerrins, 7 November 1942 (Palm Island-1942-3), MSCK.
84. Ibid.
85. Hanlon, E.M. quoted in 'Brave Nuns.' *Cairns Post*, November 12, 1940, 3.
86. Gribble, E.R. to Bishop Shevill, October 21, 1946 (Australian Board of Missions, Further Records 1873-1978, MLMSS 4503 Add On 1822, Box 9(69), G8), Mitchell Library, Sydney.
87. "John." Interview with author.
88. Davis, Albert to Atkinson, May 13, 1937 (PHD, 1935/0251, Cons 1003), SROWA.
89. Huelin, Frederick to Mother Margaret, July 22, 1937 (PHD, 1935/0251, Cons 1003), SROWA.
90. Musso, L.A. to Atkinson, March 4, 1941 (PHD, 1940/0390, Cons 1003), SROWA; Carroll, H. to Atkinson, February 26 and March 9, 1948 and Ross, R. to Atkinson, June 24, 1948 (PHD, 1946/0875, Cons 1003), SROWA.
91. 'St John of God and the Aboriginal Missions,' 1954 (2.68A), SSJGB.
92. Moroney, 'Reminiscences.'
93. Pan, Eileen. 1997. 'Pray for Us.' In *The Telling of Stories* ed. Peter Bibby, 60.

94. Ibid.
95. Puertollano, 'These Were the Girls,' 53.
96. Ibid., 54.
97. Henschke to Kerrins, April 11, 1944 (Prov Corr, NT Darwin 1944), MSCK.
98. Henschke to Kerrins, August 23, 1944 (Prov Corr, NT Darwin 1944), MSCK.
99. Henschke to Kerrins, December 14, 1943 (Prov Corr, NT Darwin 1943), MSCK.
100. 'Channel Island' in *Smile of Mary*, Christimas 1944.
101. Bachelier, Father. 1959. 'They Received the Mission Cross.' *The Annal of Our Lady of the Sacred Heart*, April 1, 101.
102. Henschke to Kerrins, March 29, 1945 (Prov Corr, NT Darwin 1945), MSCK.

CHAPTER 7

Births, Betrothals, and 'Bad' Behaviour

The expectation that leprosarium patients would undergo unproven and odious therapies, provide their labour for little or no pay, and submit to attempts to inculcate them with Christianity and Western culture might be seen as one layer of control over their lives, even if unenforced and in the benevolent, healing spirit of their carers. But the more rigid controls related to the essential function of the leprosarium—the prevention of the spread of disease—were set down as state laws or institutional rules. By stripping patients of their freedom of movement and access to home and family, leprosarium detention was the most restrictive of these. Others were rules to segregate the sexes, remove newborns from the parents, and orderly behaviour. This chapter explores what these rules meant for patients and for the staff and administrators who implemented them, and how patients accommodated or resisted them. It examines this aspect of leprosarium life at Derby, Fantome Island, Channel Island, and East Arm, the mainland institution that replaced the latter.

Sexuality and Family

On entering the leprosaria, patients became subject to strict practices restricting their sexuality and opportunities for parenting. In the imposition of these policies, government health authorities followed international conventions aimed at protecting the health of both the public and

C. Robson, *Missionary Women, Leprosy and Indigenous Australians, 1936–1986*, https://doi.org/10.1007/978-3-031-05796-0_7

the patients. They were upheld by the Catholic nursing Sisters for this reason and in the interests of promoting Christian morality and maintaining social order. Resistance by patients to these regulations reinforced preconceptions of Indigenous people as irresponsible with regard to their sexuality and health. Yet their resistance also invoked a change in policy to allow marriages. Marriages were an attempt by religious and state authorities to contain sexual relations within the contemporary Christian framework of fidelity and domesticity and symbolised the attainment of moral and social advancement under the guiding hand of the Catholic staff, thus mirroring the reforming agenda of Indigenous missions. The removal of babies born at the leprosaria, however, prevented patients from ever fully realising the Catholic family ideal. This practice, together with their exclusion from decisions concerning the future welfare of these children, signified that as Indigenous leprosy sufferers, they were perceived as unfit for parenthood. The children, as with their parents, were a problem group best managed by Catholic religious Sisters, in the view of government authorities. Taking responsibility for fostering out the children facilitated expansion of missionary aims outside the gates of the leprosaria and took no account of the parents' own family connections and religious affiliations. At times, this role outweighed the resources available to Catholic women's religious communities, resulting in tragedy and leading to the inescapable conclusion that provisions for the health care and well-being of Indigenous children were sometimes better inside than outside the leprosarium.

At all Australian leprosaria attempts were made to maintain sexual segregation for all patients through the provision of separate quarters for the men and women.[1] Even patients who were admitted along with relatives of the opposite sex, such as fathers and their daughters, were segregated.[2] Healthy spouses and children were prohibited from coming to live in detention. Work and leisure activities in the leprosarium were also usually undertaken in separate groups. Women and men sat separately "at meals, in church and at movie showings."[3] Only in situations in which patients were under more intense surveillance, such as concert performances, was this rule relaxed.

Health authorities were not so much concerned about the possibility of sexual intercourse itself, but the consequential birth of children who, through close physical contact with their parents, were considered to have a high probability of contracting leprosy.[4] Another issue was the mother's health as pregnancy and childbirth could compromise the health of a leprosy sufferer and result in acute illness and even death.[5] At most leprosaria in Australia and overseas, sexual segregation policies were enforced but, in some parts of the world, they were relaxed on condition that male patients submit to sterilisation procedures.[6]

Religious staff objected to sexual relations between the patients for moral reasons. On her arrival at Fantome Island, Mother Peter complained to Bishop Ryan, "My Lord, we find the moral condition of our poor people in a deplorable state. The building accommodation is temporarily inadequate. The sexes are intermixed."[7] A similar situation greeted the Channel Island Sisters on their arrival in 1943, causing the same anxiety. Extramarital sexual relationships in the leprosarium were, for the Sisters, a sign of low self-esteem and such behaviour demanded their immediate attention. At both leprosaria, there was protest by some of the male patients when, after further buildings were constructed, the women were finally separated from the men.[8] It was perhaps an overly optimistic Mother Peter who tried to console the men with a gift each of new pyjamas and a salutary speech by the superintendent.[9]

Mother Peter did not condemn outright the idea of sexual relations between the patients, however, for, within a few months of her arrival in 1940, when the Queensland Health Department refused a request for marriages to be allowed, she remarked: "We were sorry to hear of their not being permitted to marry as there are some to whom we would have proposed such."[10] Sexual relationships within the sacred institution of a Christian marriage were clearly acceptable if attempts to stop them unregulated failed. Perhaps she realised immediately the impracticability of the ban on marriages and may have also seen marriage as a way of preventing promiscuity and the consequential sexual rivalry. Fr Damien, the late superintendent of Molokai leprosarium had "advised that faithful husbands and wives should be allowed to go to the settlement, he permitted marriages between lepers previously unmarried, and found these measures led to contentment and improved morality."[11] It was a philosophy that almost certainly would be known to Mother Peter, being one of a generation of Catholic Sisters who studied Damien's life in detail.

Concerns by the Channel Island missionaries over sexual advances made by male patients reveal racial undertones implicit in the Catholic missionary paradigm. When the Sisters' attempts to rein in their behaviour led to patient protest in 1946, the matron, Mother Michaeline complained to government officials,

> The black girls – only children. The half-castes have been trying to take them for wives. We have never spoken to the half-castes themselves about it, but we have spoken to the children and told them to keep out of their way. They are the children in the dormitory.[12]

Sexual advances towards the young Indigenous girls by European or part-European men was unacceptable behaviour on moral grounds for government and church authorities, and was particularly galling for the Catholic missionaries to witness what they took to be the moral decline of their protégés, the Bathurst Island mission girls. Fr William Henschke, like Mother Michaeline, thought it was the girls' responsibility to refuse the men's advances. "I spoke strongly to the Catholics and told them they should be ashamed of themselves… I told the blackies they have an immortal soul, are not animals and if the men want to sin with them, to refuse…"[13]

His expectation was that the girls, having had a mission education, would defend their own Christian virtue by repelling the men's sexual advances and thereby act as guardians for correct behaviour between the sexes. As historian Tony Scanlon has argued, it was an approach utilised typically by Catholic missionaries to promote Christian sexual morality among Indigenous Australians, particularly in cases involving European men.[14] The mission dynamics of moral mentor and innocent child of the bush, facilitating the inculcation of Christian moral principles, were fractured in the leprosarium by the intrusion of others—patients from diverse backgrounds, with varying attitudes to sexuality.

The sexual predation of young girls by men continued to be seen as a major problem for religious and government authorities. The Sisters shielded the girls in quarters close to their convents, and at some distance from the patients' quarters.[15] The convents had been positioned to be out-of-bounds to patients—designated "clean areas," indicating that they were free of disease—but in reality, the threat of sexual violation outweighed that of bacterial contamination. Indigenous law relating to sexual and marital practices lost much of their force in the leprosarium as the security and guidance of the family and wider kinship network were mostly left behind or disrupted by the institutional system of familial segregation. In their place, the Sisters became the moral guardians when neither physical barriers nor rejection by the girls were found to be effective.

Despite all measures to maintain separation between the men and women, it was impossible for staff to prevent the patients from conducting clandestine sexual liaisons. Long-term romantic partnerships were forged, many of which resulted in the birth of children. As men staked claims over the hearts of particular women, the formation of what one government official called the "eternal triangle" led to many a *crime passionnel*.[16] The Sisters patched up injuries inflicted as a result of such conflicts, and on several occasions, the violence worsened to the point of life-threatening blows.[17] The frequent physical violence was a constant worry to the Sisters and lay authorities. Believing it to be rooted in competition for the women's affections, the Sisters tried various means to divert the men's attention away from the opposite sex to other activities, including, as already mentioned, introducing the orchestra at the Derby leprosarium.

By the late 1940s, patients with leprosy were permitted to marry, mainly to keep the peace. After a particularly intense skirmish between some patients at Fantome Island, the medical officer successfully appealed to the health department to allow test permits for marriage, arguing, "Patients would lead a more normal life and most of the trouble would be avoided if they were allowed to marry."[18] The perceived benefits of marriage for the harmony of the leprosarium can also be found in correspondence by staff members, such as Sister Benedicta who advocated marriage between two patients "From the point of view of the morality, general health and discipline of the Settlement…"[19]

The earliest marriages were organised according to European protocol and without reference to patients' own traditions. Couples required the matron's recommendation and, under Indigenous protection legislation, the consent of the Director of Native Affairs (or equivalent officer). Successful candidates were usually young, single, and in long-standing monogamous relationships. Staff recommendations contained comments such as, "Since their childhood, they promised to be faithful to each other" and "they have been together since 1939."[20] To partake in a wedding ceremony, the couples had to be Christian and of the same denomination, so some had to undertake religious instruction and receive the sacraments beforehand. Many conversions were to Catholicism due to the influence of the Catholic staff and chaplains. Weddings were the first stages of the creation of new Catholic families.

But, in glibly brokering these European-style marriages, staff neglected to consider the consequences for the societies left behind by leprosarium patients. Social obligations to the clan and family, particularly for young women, persisted despite the physical separation of the patient from her home country. In 1953, for example, a twelve-year-old girl from Liverpool River was abducted from Channel Island by her intended husband and his relatives. About a week later, the party was located, and the girl returned to the leprosarium while the men were exiled to the Philip Creek Reserve.[21]

The status of marriage brought with it certain privileges. No longer considered in need of the Sisters' protection, wives left the dormitories and set up house with their husbands in their own cottages in the "married compounds," allowing them more privacy and independence. The couples were encouraged to create European-style domiciles. They cultivated vegetable and flower gardens and cooked their own meals, rather than dine from the common kitchen. Domestic pride and competence, revealed in clean linen, neat flower beds and swept floors, seemed, as with commitment to marriage itself, evidence of successful assimilation to lives of Christian morality and respectability. To all appearances, the married couples were the responsible patients, entrusted by the Sisters with keeping an eye on the young patients or called on in emergencies.[22] The extension of the right to marry led to patients' assuming the kind of "civic pride" discussed by historian Warwick Anderson in his study of the Culion leprosarium.[23] In Australia, as with the Philippines, the rights implicit in this role, however, could never be truly exercised by those, who by virtue of their race or disease, would continually be subject to discriminatory practices (Fig. 7.1).

A similar paradox operated with respect to preparation for family life. If European homemaking was held up as an ideal to which young patients were taught to aspire, its implicit purpose, of raising children, could never be fulfilled. Infants were removed from their parents immediately after the birth and prevented from having any further physical contact. Of all the terrible experiences remembered by former leprosarium patients and the nursing Sisters, the removal of the children stands out as the most traumatic.[24] The policy, implemented by Australian health departments until the late 1960s, was intended to protect the child from contracting leprosy through parental contact.[25] Yet the fact remains that for Indigenous people everywhere, it was one of many justifications for denying them the right to raise their own children.[26] Only if patients were discharged would there be a chance of reunion with their children. Until the late 1950s, factors such as the high death rate, ineffective drug therapy, and strict criteria for discharge, made reunions between patients and their

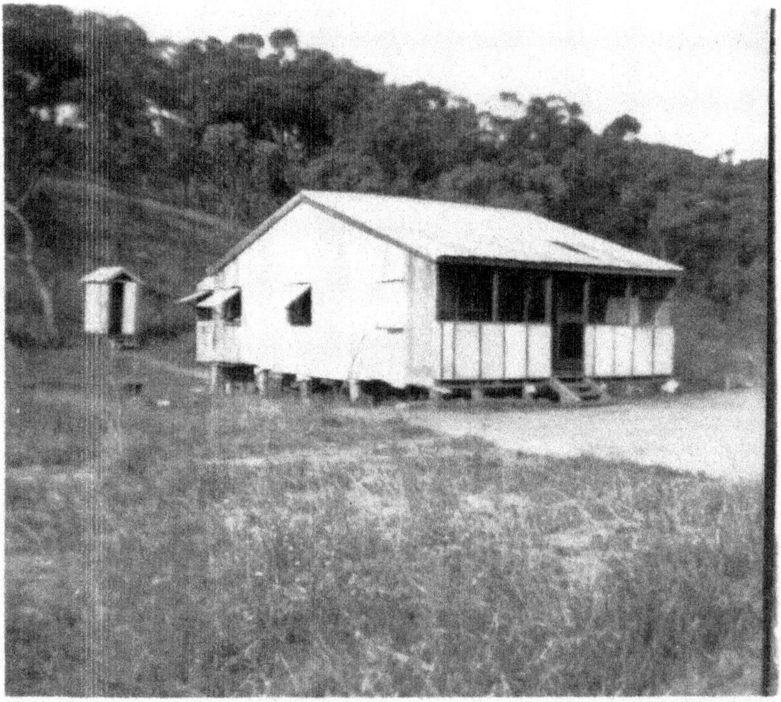

Fig. 7.1 'House built by patient for himself and wife, mainly out of scrap iron and timber, Lazaret, Fantome Island,' late 1940s (Queensland State Archives)

offspring extremely unlikely. The babies, then, were viewed by authorities as orphans, and responsibility for their welfare officially lay with state health and Indigenous affairs departments.

Various interests were at work in determining the appropriate custody for patients' newborns. Health authorities considered them to be a problem group who, without careful upbringing and continued surveillance, posed a public danger in a more intense form of bureaucratic fears around growing numbers of 'mixed-race' Indigenous children throughout the first half of the twentieth century.[27] At risk, in both cases, was a healthy white Australia, the former through their potential for spreading disease and the latter, through racial degeneration. Since signs of leprosy may not be evident for many years, health departments maintained that "they require repeated examination over several years and must not be permitted to be removed from medical observation during childhood or youth."[28] This factor limited the eligibility of potential Indigenous foster families since few communities were adequately provided with medical or nursing services. Furthermore, fears of latent disease in the children deterred many families from taking them on. Governments therefore turned to the support of the Catholic mission Sisters, as they had for the care of the parents.

Usually, leprosarium babies were fostered out to Catholic orphanages or to Catholic missions where suitable Indigenous foster families were found and the supervision of missionary nursing Sisters could be ensured. Babies born at Derby leprosarium were habitually transferred to Beagle Bay mission; Channel Island babies to Bathurst Island; and Fantome Island babies to Palm Island.[29] Raised as members of Catholic mission communities, the children extended the thread connecting their families with the Sisters and their Church. For some, this link was generations old, but for others, it began with a diagnosis of leprosy. In the latter cases, the children's upbringing in the Catholic mission environment marked a departure from the traditions of their parents and assimilation into the life of the local Indigenous Catholic community.

Appropriate care for the infants was sometimes impossible to procure. In their first few months, these babies were often of low birthweight and frail health, and prone to diseases such as influenza and pneumonia. They consequently required intensive supervision, particularly in the immediate post-natal stage, with frequent feeds, regular health checks, and monitoring of their environment.[30] In some cases, neonates remained in the care of the leprosarium Sisters until they had gained weight and improved in health, but as priority was usually given to their prompt removal, the more common procedure was to transfer them to the local hospital for a few weeks before fostering them out.[31] However at Derby Native Hospital in the 1940s, resources were overstretched. The sole nurse, in addition to her normal sixty-one patients, was expected to care for three babies born around the same time at the leprosarium.[32] Rather than send them to the smaller and more generously staffed District Hospital for Europeans, the Health Department asked the SSJG Sisters to find foster care for them. The Holy Child Orphanage in Broome could not accept them as they did not have the necessary staff for the special attention required, but Sister Gertrude Greene, after considerable difficulty, found foster mothers in the Broome area for a total of four infants.[33]

Several months later, Dr Milne, the local doctor, inspected the camps where two of the babies were living. He reported immediately to Cecil Cook, the Western Australia Health Commissioner: "there is no water or sanitation. About 10–12 persons live in this 'camp' in conditions of filth, vermin and overcrowding which almost defeats the senses.…I cannot too strongly recommend the removal of these two babies from their present surroundings and beg that something be done to demolish the so-called 'Camp.'"[34] The Commissioner asked Sister Gertrude if she could find some other women to take charge of the children, but nothing was done and, by the following April, two of the babies, a boy and girl, were dead, both from pneumonia.[35] Of the little boy, the Coroner stated, that the foster parents were not suitable and "did not appreciate the proper nursing of the baby."[36] The girl was a "victim of neglect and indifference on part of foster mother" and was "admitted to hospital suffering from scabies, malnutrition, stomatitis, bronchopneumonia."[37]

These cases were not unique, nor were such tragedies confined to offspring of the Derby patients. Although the infants may have developed life-threatening conditions even in the most ideal environment, they clearly did not receive the care they deserved. The biological parents, stripped of their rights as nurturers and providers, were also let down. In all probability, the infants would have fared better had they remained in the leprosarium where, even with the risk of contracting leprosy, their welfare and longevity were more assured. But, as this anecdote reinforces, health departments were not prepared to take this chance, such was the fear of leprosy.

The Derby crisis of the post-war 1940s reflects the paucity of nursing services to remotely situated Indigenous people. The difficulty in obtaining lay nurses for this kind of work was to some extent ameliorated by the willingness of nursing Sisters from various missionary organisations to fill the gap, but in this period, there were still too few. Many Sisters belonging to the small SSJG Kimberley community, such as Sister Gertrude, were approaching old age and few vocations were forthcoming to replace them. It was, at times, then, with misplaced confidence that the leprosarium babies, like ticking time bombs, were gratefully passed by government health departments into the Sisters' hands.

The infants' deaths did nothing to change the practices of the Western Australia Health Department, as two years later, its officers could again be found appealing to the SSJG Sisters to find foster mothers for more leprosarium babies.[38] However, Sister Gertrude, remorseful over her self-confessed failure in the affair, proposed a plan to Dr Cook to increase nursing services in Derby: Derby Native Hospital could be put under the charge of her congregation of Sisters who would then train local Indigenous girls to be nurses.[39] In 1952, the necessary permission to do so was granted.[40]

It appears that some patients without affiliations with the Catholic Church were unhappy about their children being fostered out to Catholic missions. To what extent this dissatisfaction prevailed cannot be assessed due to the lack of sources directly conveying patients' views but some evidence from the 1940s can be found in the documents of visiting missionaries to Derby and of welfare officers dispatched to Channel Island. In the Kimberley in this period, United Aborigines Mission (UAM) and Presbyterian missionaries battled the health department to have babies discharged into their care in cases where the parents originated from, or had connections with, their missions.[41] A UAM missionary told the health department that one couple "both individually appealed to us to do what we could to get them [sic] back as they want their child to be brought up Protestant."[42] Sectarian rivalry may have played a part in such requests, but there is no reason to doubt that patients wanted their children raised at their home missions, particularly if they themselves had been discharged back, as in the case of one father from Kunmunya on whose behalf Presbyterian missionaries petitioned in 1948.[43] In this period, there were few avenues other than visiting missionaries through which Indigenous patients, especially women, could express such grievances.

Discipline

The detention policy and strict regimes within the leprosarium would always be met with powerful resistance by some Indigenous people, regardless of attempts to soften their impact by the religious staff. If removal from home to institutional confinement was not reason enough for discontent, then the leprosarium itself was, with its restrictions on personal freedom, suppression of normal social and cultural customs, and the regular grind of the painful therapeutic regime. Absconding, unregulated sex, fighting and dissension continued to occur throughout the periods in which the institutions operated, deplored by staff and governments for the threats they posed to the core objective of secure and harmonious isolation. For governments experienced in managing the institutional confinement of Indigenous people, these violations stemmed from primitive yearnings and were to be dealt with the same way, irrespective of the fact that the leprosaria were not Indigenous reserves. Sometimes harsh, sometimes gentle, disciplinary measures by both lay and religious staff were almost always infused with the paternalism that typified interracial relations in this period. At the different institutions, the inclusion of patients with varied racial and social backgrounds complicated and challenged efforts to maintain compliance and internal social order.

The offence most feared by authorities was absconding, in the knowledge that some patients would do anything to return to their land and families. Island sites made escape difficult, but not impossible, and many people absconded, usually in groups, and sometimes with the assistance of friends outside the leprosarium.[44] Some escapees were never found, perhaps having died on the arduous journey home. Not all absconders intended to leave the leprosarium permanently, but to fulfil a cultural obligation to visit friends and family.[45] Some groups left as a form of protest, while others in mainland institutions slipped away for a drink in town.[46] But all were considered serious risks to public health and police were called to locate and return the patients.

Policies to maintain disciplinary control borrowed heavily from regulations for government Indigenous reserves, particularly Queensland and Western Australia.[47] Male superintendents were from the same pool of personnel on these reserves and, as in those places, were expected to maintain order in the leprosaria, especially over the male patients, by preventing fights and breaches of rules, many of which arose from provocative policies such as sexual segregation and the blending of people from traditionally oppositional groups.[48] At Derby, male superintendents and, later, their assistants, were continually on staff and always accompanied by their wives, who were given some responsibility over the female patients. They were not Protectors of Aboriginals, and, under health regulations, they could act only under the authority of the relevant medical officer on an area gazetted as a lazaret. Furthermore, some patients were not classified under state acts as "Aboriginal" and therefore even outside the leprosarium were not legally subject to this kind of control. Nevertheless, at Fantome Island until the late 1940s, and at Derby throughout its period of operation, superintendents took charge of disciplinary matters. After the departure of Superintendent Julian from Fantome Island in

1947, disciplinary control was overseen by the Palm Island superintendent. The latter was a Protector, but in theory, if not in practice, his control over the patients was relinquished from 1949 when all patients were granted exemption from the Queensland Aboriginals Act by the state government in the unsuccessful attempt to qualify leprosarium patients for the Commonwealth invalid pension.

Another policy inspired by state Indigenous regulations at Fantome Island and Derby was the formation of small police forces drawn from the patient populations, and operating under orders of the superintendents.[49] Patient police forces were also in use concurrently at overseas leprosaria, including Kalaupapa (Hawaii) and Culion (Philippines).[50] They were especially useful in keeping order at Fantome Island from the late 1940s after Julian's departure although one former patient attests to their turning a blind eye to some breaches of the rules.[51] Boasting uniforms and batons and led by a "sergeant" they were to some extent a show of unconsummated power. As well as a deterrent, they were also an example of ideal inmate behaviour, rewarded with the prestige of their positions, sanctioned use of weapons and smart apparel. As Anna Haebich has discussed of police at Moore River Settlement in Western Australia, their place in an institution was uncertain, having neither the confidence of other inmates nor the status of white staff.[52] The term 'police' was avoided by leprosarium authorities, as if there was an awareness of the illegitimacy of this practice. At Fantome Island, they were "orderlies" and at Derby, they "call[ed] them leaders, never used to call them police boys."[53]

Another component of the Indigenous reserve discipline system was the jail. Until the mid-1950s there was no legal provision in health regulations for confining patients in a cell, but every leprosarium hospital included a locked ward, and staff members were authorised to restrain patients who were believed at risk of absconding. It is not clear how long people were left in this state. Certainly, some presented ongoing difficulties for the Derby superintendent who in 1937 asked for, and was granted, a set of chains for restraining patients.[54] Unofficially, patients displaying a range of other undesirable behaviours, such as psychoses and sexual immorality were also physically restrained or confined.[55]

Still one more practice that aligns the system at Fantome Island with the Queensland reserve system was the interception of patients' mail. Incoming and outgoing correspondence between patients and the patient welfare organisation, the Relatives and Friends Association (RFA), was passed to the Palm Island superintendent who then passed it to the Department of Native Affairs without it having reached its intended recipients, including one that was handed in by one of the nursing Sisters.[56] Among them were letters written by the RFA secretary to two patients, in which the Department was severely criticised for conditions at the leprosarium. According to the Deputy Director, their contents, if exposed would have "a serious adverse effect on the harmony and well-being of Fantome Island."[57]

Channel Island was the only leprosarium where the replication of reserve policies was not discernible, possibly because some patients were European. The administration relied more on the presence of authority, mostly in the form of the superintendent, to deter patients from disobedience or recalcitrance in the absence of a legally valid system of penalties.[58] However, Brother Carter found the legal constraints to his power frustrating and applied to the Department of Native Affairs to be appointed a Protector of Aboriginals, stating that since he "has to adjudicate in tribal squabbles his position would be more authoritative."[59] The Department turned down his request. The island had no patient police. When patients caused trouble, the Northern Territory Police were called in to "threaten the natives with some action if these troubles continued... It was realised by all here that such threats were idle, but they had the effect of temporarily abating the nuisances at Channel Island."[60]

The interpretation by superintendents of their roles varied depending on the individual and the influence of competing sources of authority. While some superintendents, such as Brother McCarthy, were reluctant to control the patients at all, and others did their best to keep the patients occupied with sports and entertainment, some individuals disregarded legal limitations and the moral rights of the patients and resorted to inhumane forms of punishment. Julian had three male patients shipped out to Curacao Island for three nights without any shelter in poor weather, a punishment customarily used for Palm Island residents. He then locked them in the cells at the lock hospital on a reduced diet. By the time "they were pleading with me," they were released.[61]

A former patient from Derby leprosarium recalled that,

> Some of the bosses were pretty rough...If you got into trouble they used to cut [the patients'] hair, make them stand there in the sun. The boss would cut it off, the police boys would help them.[62]

The leprosarium Sisters viewed the patients as children in need of firm parental guidance. Mother Peter of Fantome Island constantly referred to her patients as "such very little ones" and "children," regardless of their ages.[63] Whether or not they were officially charged with the responsibility of disciplining the patients, they saw themselves as the patients' rightful 'parents.' Displays of brutality by the superintendent invoked the Derby Sisters' compassion and undermined their agenda of nurturing a genteel Christian citizenry. In recalling the treatment described above, the ex-patient said: "The nuns used to go crazy, they were against it…"[64]

In other situations, the Sisters themselves imposed harsh disciplinary measures. After Julian left Fantome Island, the Sisters dealt with violent outbursts and sexual transgressions by locking patients in their quarters or at the hospital, presumably with the assistance of the patient police force.[65] Allegations of brutal punishments by Sisters at Channel Island were made by a recently discharged part-descent patient, Nida Cahill, in 1946. If the allegations were taken seriously, the result is unknown.[66]

From the early 1950s, the maintenance of peace and social order in the leprosaria seems to have become more challenging to staff than earlier. Absconding continued and violence increased, and became, in some instances, more extreme. Higher patient numbers in Western Australia and Northern Territory (approximately 250 and 200 respectively in 1954) was probably a contributing factor. Northern Territory welfare officers attributed disciplinary problems to boredom, arguing that insufficient staff and funds had been supplied to keep the whole patient population occupied with work or recreation. Effective drugs may also have made patients feel better and therefore more restless.

For health departments in Western Australia and Northern Territory, suggestions of more recreational facilities were inadequate for managing serious patient infringements. They wanted to restrain and punish the patient and deter others from following their example. Officials in this period became more conscious of the need to do so legally, and without excessive brutality, especially in the Territory, where public scrutiny had increased in the years after the World War II. Furthermore, the government's new Welfare Branch favoured a softly-softly approach. Chains had once been used to restrain patients but could no longer be justified. Health Acts made no provision for restraining patients unless they tried to abscond. In 1954, the Health Act of Western Australia was amended to include the *Derby Leprosarium Regulations* and the definition of "detention" was broadened to include confinement in locked quarters within the leprosarium.[67] They also spelt out the categories of patients deemed eligible for this treatment:

> A mental patient or other patient whose conduct is likely to cause injury to other persons or damage to property in the institution, may be confined to detention quarters or otherwise forcibly restrained as necessary.[68]

In addition, patients convicted of serious crimes and given jail sentences could serve their time in the leprosarium cell, as public jail wardens refused to guard prisoners afflicted with leprosy.[69]

In 1957, after Channel Island was replaced with a new leprosarium on the mainland at East Arm, a spate of serious spear fights and other violent episodes including an attack on a Sister, led the Director of Health, A.H. Humphry, to ask the advice of his counterparts in Western Australia and Queensland on how their leprosarium patients were "legally disciplined."[70]

> We could take things into our own hands and lock them up without legal authority, but Darwin suffers from a surfeit of reporters (mainly to interview V.I.P.s travelling to and from Australia) who would only be too pleased to make a good story out of 'ill-treatment' of 'poor lepers'.[71]

The Queensland Director-General of Health, Abraham Fryberg, replied that with Fantome Island's small population, few problems arose and so harsher penalties were not required—a strange statement coming soon after a patient had been imprisoned on Palm Island for murdering another patient.[72] The Western Australia Health Commissioner, Linley Henzell, supplied Humphry with a copy of the Derby regulations and an invitation to look over the new detention cell, a central concrete structure with a corrugated iron roof and verandahs enclosed with steel mesh.[73]

Although keen to follow Derby's example, Humphry could find little support for a jail, and East Arm used its isolation block, normally reserved for patients at risk of absconding or suffering from psychoses, as punishment. The welfare officers thought a cell inappropriate for a medical institution, and legal advisors doubted there was any legitimate right to confine patients on grounds of undesirable behaviour.[74] The superintendent preferred milder penalties such as withholding tobacco or permission to watch movies.[75] Patients were upset that absconding and throwing spears might lead to time in the cell. One patient, aware that cell

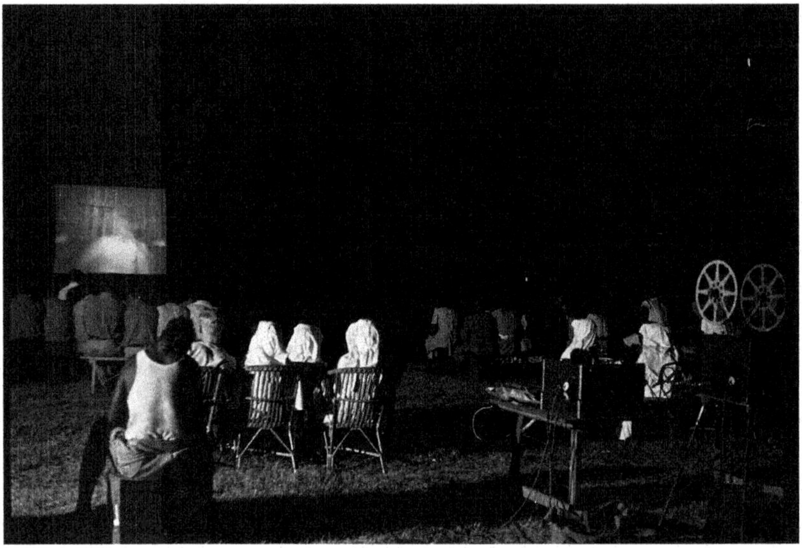

Fig. 7.2 'Nurses and patients at outdoor movie show, Derby Leprosarium 1948' (Stuart Gore Collection, State Library of Western Australia)

confinement was not legal, complained that Mother Benedicta and the superintendent "alway take the law into their own liking" (Fig. 7.2).[76]

At East Arm and Derby, existing laws were liberally interpreted to allow for punishing undesirable behaviour.[77] The former relied on the *Leprosy Ordinance* (NT), under which patients could be restrained to prevent a recurrence of absconding, or attempting to abscond, from the leprosarium, to confine patients in the isolation block.[78] It was used to lock away patients for acts of violence but as these usually occurred after breaking out of the leprosarium and obtaining liquor, their imprisonment could be justified as a means of preventing further absconding.[79]

Patient Protest

Indigenous patients, particularly those with minimal experience of European society, had few opportunities to petition for change to conditions in the leprosaria. Alison Bashford has argued that avenues of protest were enabled in multiracial leprosaria (such as Peel Island prior to 1940), "partly because the space and experience of isolation-as-leper was shared with whites."[80] Similarly, in the northern leprosaria, complaints about conditions and patient rights were also more often—but not exclusively—initiated by part-European or European patients, being more aware of their rights and ways to assert them. Nevertheless, Indigenous patients did at times both participate in, and initiate, various forms of contestation.

European or part-European patients at Channel and Fantome Islands protested their subjection to the authority of the Catholic nursing Sisters, indicating their belief that lay staff would be less oppressive. In 1946, patients walked off Channel Island to form a deputation to the Chief Medical Officer with a raft of complaints. Before leaving, someone scrawled on a wall "Out with Campion and her mob!"[81] A subsequent investigation commissioned by the Northern Territory government administration, in which staff and patients were interviewed, revealed that one focus of their complaints was the Catholic staff and the desire to replace them with a lay matron and curator as in former years. It concluded that although several Indigenous patients were among the protesters, the main perpetrators were four male European patients as well as several part-descent patients of both sexes who resented attempts by the Sisters to control their sexual and spiritual lives.[82]

On Fantome Island in 1949, a part-European patient, Jack Harrison, aired his grievances during a visit to the leprosarium by an official party including the Queensland Home Secretary. As related to Anglican minister, Rev. E.R. Gribble by the medical officer, he

> began by saying that he was a free man, had voted at elections, paid taxes etc and he now wanted to make complaints as to the treatment at the leprosarium. He said 'letters from my family are opened, parcels they send are opened, and I am forever being asked to join the R.C. Church. I want to be removed to Peel Island.'[83]

In both this speech and the demands of the Northern Territory patients, and in other letters, there was an appeal to citizenship rights and the rejection of the paternalism characteristic of the Sisters' management.[84] Requests were made for transfer to Peel Island where lay management, better conditions and access to medical care were viewed as a means to restore dignity and maximise chances for recovery. Implicitly, part-European and European patients did not want to be treated as Indigenous patients.

But neither did the Sisters want them as patients, regarding them as troublesome and corrupting influences on the 'Aboriginal' inmates. Although the report of the Northern Territory inquiry recommended replacement of the religious Sisters and Brother with lay personnel, the federal Minister for Health, Nick McKenna, became convinced by their religious superiors that it was actually the patients of European descent who were the problem and it was they who should be removed.[85] Not one leprosarium in the Commonwealth, however, would accept the mixed descent patients, with the exception of Derby which admitted one patient, originally from Western Australia. With his return, the radicalism of the two island institutions seemed to have been transferred to the more insular Derby leprosarium. The Derby superintendent appealed for his return to Channel Island as "his influence among the natives and other half-caste inmates is fostering an attitude of indiscipline, suspicion and resentment hitherto completely unknown at Derby."[86]

In the early 1950s, patient activism was boosted by the support of advocates outside the leprosarium. The patient welfare group, the RFA agitated on behalf of the people at Peel and Fantome Islands, provided material support to the patients and worked to lessen the social stigma of leprosy. Its members pressed government for improved conditions and medical care, as well as the relaxation of discharge criteria, and circulated its newsletter, the *Moreton Star* to patients, alerting them to their rights. In 1951, a patient wrote to the E. Hinton, the RFA Secretary, expressing his "joy to know that there is someone who is doing their uttermost for us."[87] The patient complained of low wages, no pensions, substandard housing, and restricted movement on the island. Poor tobacco was equated with "what Captain Cook has trade [sic] with the natives of Australia to take the country away from us."[88] He blamed the government for these problems, but not the Sisters as "they have their instructions to go by and we know they simply got to carry it out"; it was the Queensland government at fault.[89] His letter was one of those intercepted by the Department of Native Affairs, and, when Hinton applied to visit Fantome Island, the patient was discharged: "To avoid a repetition of untrue and libellous statements made by this man it is hoped that his transfer to Palm Island has been effected before Mr Hinton's arrival."[90] Thus, the pattern continued of removing refractory patients, of believing, or preferring to believe, that the problem was with the patient, not the place.

In the 1940s and 1950s, patients could seldom rely on the religious staff for support in their battles for better conditions.[91] Fantome Island's Sr St Nérée who had passed the abovementioned patient's letter and a copy of the *Moreton Star* to the Palm Island superintendent opposed such dissension, in particular the criticism of discharge policies of the Director-General of Health, aligning it to blasphemy:

> This paper, "Moreton Star" criticises authority, which came from God. 'Thou wouldst have no power at all over me ere it not given thee from above.' St John, Ch.XIX, 11.[92]

In an enduring reference to the New Testament, the patients were expected to bear their crosses stoically.

For this reason, inquiries such as at Channel Island in 1946, which brought outsiders with authority into the leprosarium to meet with the patients, were important means of bringing attention to institutional deficiencies. The interviews exposed the practice of employing Indigenous men to chop wood for no pay whatsoever, the scarcity of medical visits, insufficient huts, the unbalanced diet and therefore a wide range of issues affecting all the patients, not just those that formed the basis of the original protest. Patient interviews at Fantome Island in the 1950s by medical officer, Morgan Gabriel also served the same purpose. These sessions seemed to be the only way to kick-start improvements but even these took time and could never compensate for the inherent deficiencies of the island sites.[93]

Notes

1. Huelin, Frederick (Under-Secretary), Memorandum: Derby Leprosarium, 13 June 1937 (Public Health Department (PHD), 1935/0251, Cons 1003), State Records Office Western Australia (SROWA); 'Rough Plan of the Leprosarium, Derby, WA, 1946–7' (Local History Collection, Leprosarium 1940–1960), Derby Local Library, Western Australia; "John" (former patient, Fantome Island Leprosarium). Interview with author. June 7, 2011. Typed transcript. Location and name confidential; Venard, Mary. 1974. *The History of the Australian Province of the Daughters of Our Lady of the Sacred Heart*. Kensington: Daughters of Our Lady of the Sacred Heart, 180.
2. Former patient "A" of Derby Leprosarium (name withheld). Interview with Christine Choo, 1992, sound recording.

3. Dunne, Sister Francis, Speech, March 8, 2002 (2.21Y), Sisters of St John of God Archives, Broome, Western Australia (SSJGB).
4. Rogers, Leonard, and Ernest Muir. 1946. *Leprosy*, third edition. Baltimore: The Williams and Wilkins Co., 129.
5. Duncan, M.E. 1993. 'An Historical and Clinical Review of the Interaction of Leprosy and Pregnancy: A Cycle to Be Broken.' *Social Science and Medicine*, 37 (4), 457; Sister Francis, Speech; Rogers, and Muir, Leprosy, 229; Poidevin, Sister Camille SJG. Interview with author. Typed transcript. Recorded at Derby, Western Australia, November 17, 2008.
6. Moran, Michelle T. 2007. *Colonising Leprosy: Imperialism and the Politics of Public Health in the United States*. Chapel Hill: University of North Carolina Press, 147–148; Rogers and Muir, *Leprosy*, 130; 'Japan's Government Compensates Leprosy Patients for Isolation Policy.' *The Lancet* 357, May 19, 2001, 1599.
7. Anderson, Mother Peter to Ryan, Bishop Hugh, March 6, 1940 (1148, Box 57, Folder 924), Townsville Cathedral Archives (TCA).
8. Venard, *History of the Australian Province*, 179–180.
9. Monthly Journal of the Our Lady Help of Christians (OLHC) at Fantome Island, March 1941 (1144, Box 57, Folder 920), TCA.
10. Ibid.
11. Rogers and Muir, *Leprosy*, 131.
12. 'Interviews by committee of inquiry-Channel Island Leprosarium,' 9 (A1928, 715/38/1 Section 3), National Archives of Australia (NAA).
13. Henschke, Father William to Gsell, Bishop F.X., September 10, 1946 (Provincial Correspondence, N.T. Darwin, 1946), Missionaries of the Sacred Heart Archives Kensington (MSCK).
14. Scanlon, Tony. 1986. '"Pure and Clean and True to Christ": Black Women and White Missionaries in the North.' *Hecate* 12 (1/2), 82.
15. Kerinaiua, Philomena. c. 2002. 'Philomena's Story.' In *So Far From Home: Oral Histories of the Stolen Generations*, ed. Lana Quall. Katherine: Diwurruwurru-jaru Aboriginal Corporation, 28; Former patient "A" of Derby Leprosarium. Interview with Christine Choo; Gabriel, Morgan. 'Report on Fantome Island, July 1956' (Item ID 714733), Queensland State Archives (QSA); "Sr Jeanne" OLSH (name withheld). Interview with author. Typed transcript. Recorded at Kensington, New South Wales, August 18, 2008.
16. Acting Secretary, Queensland Department of Native Affairs (DNA), Memo, November 16, 1944 (Director of Native Affairs Office, 1A/65, PART 1, Correspondence, Aboriginal and Torres Strait Islander, ID ITM501855), QSA.
17. "Sr Helen" OLSH (name withheld). Interview with author. Typed transcript. Recorded at Kensington, NSW, August 18, 2008.

18. Reye, Eric. 'Report,' February 15, 1946 (Director of Native Affairs Office, 3A/157, Correspondence, Aboriginal and Torres Strait Islander, ID ITM505023), QSA.
19. Carroll, Sister Benedicta to O'Loughlin, Bishop John, May 31, 1956 (B140, Missionaries of the Sacred Heart Archives, Darwin (MSCD).
20. St Nérée, Sr to Queensland Minister for Health and Home Affairs, February 11, 1948 and Medical Officer to Director, July 8, 1946, both at (3A/157, ITM505023), QSA.
21. Elphinstone, Dr J.J. to Superintendent of Police, Darwin, October 5, 1953 (E51, 1959/532), NAA.
22. Former patient "John." Interview with author; Former patient, Fantome Island. (JCU ID 521, Parts 1 & 2, North Queensland Oral History Project), James Cook University; Former patient "B" of Derby Leprosarium (name withheld). Interview with Christine Choo, 1992, sound recording, State Library of Western Australia.
23. Anderson, Warwick. 2006. *Colonial Pathologies: American Tropical Medicine, Race and Hygiene in the Philippines*. Durham and London: Duke University Press, 172.
24. Anderson, John. 2005. 'Hidden from the World: Palm Man Looks Back on Tough Days as Member of an Island Leper Colony.' *Townsville Bulletin*, November 17, 11; Sister Camille, Interview with author, "Sister Helen," Interview with author, Duford, Sister Paule. Interview with Siobhan McHugh (Siobhan McHugh Collection of Australian Social History. Sound recording, 198–?, ORAL TRC 2761/5), National Library of Australia.
25. Rogers and Muir, *Leprosy*, 131.
26. Haebich, Ann. 2000. *Broken Circles: Fragmenting Indigenous Families 1800–2000*. Fremantle: Fremantle Arts Centre Press, 374.
27. McGregor, Russell. 1998. *Imagined Destinies: Aboriginal Australians and the Doomed Race Theory 1880–1939*. Carlton: Melbourne University Press, 136–138.
28. Cook, Cecil (Western Australia Commissioner of Public Health). Memo, September 10, 1946 (PHD, 1946/0875, Cons 1003), SROWA.
29. Kettle, Ellen. 1991. *Health Services in the Northern Territory: A History 1824–1970*, volume two. Darwin: North Australia Research Unit, 54; Sister Camille. Interview with author.
30. Carmody, Mother Margaret to Stitfold, H.T (Under-Secretary), August 27, 1946 (PHD, 1946/0875, Cons 1003), SROWA; Howell, Matron to Cook, 5 December 1947 (PHD, 1946/0875, Cons 1003), SROWA.
31. Western Australia Commissioner of Native Affairs (WACNA) to Cook, November 5, 1947 (PHD, 1946/0875, Cons 1003), SROWA.
32. Howell, Matron to WACNA, December 5, 1947 (PHD, 1946/0875, Cons 1003), SROWA.

33. Mother Margaret to Stitfold, August 27, 1946 and Sr Gertrude Greene to Stitfold, February 24, 1948 and May 28, 1948, all at (PHD, 1946/0875, Cons 1003), SROWA.
34. Dr Milne quoted in letter from Cook to WACNA, October 11, 1948 (PHD 1946/0875, Cons 1003), SROWA.
35. Cook to Sr Gertrude, October 13, 1948 and Milne to Cook, March 15, 1949 and April 5, 1949 all in (PHD 1946/0875, Cons 1003), SROWA.
36. The Coroner to Cook, May 2, 1949 (PHD 1946/0875, Cons 1003), SROWA.
37. Milne to Cook, April 5, 1949 (PHD 1946/0875, Cons 1003), SROWA.
38. Deputy Commissioner of Public Health to WACNA, November 21, 1951 (PHD 1946/0875, Cons 1003), SROWA.
39. Sr Gertrude to Cook, April 10, 1949 (PHD 1946/0875, Cons 1003), SROWA.
40. Sisters of St John of God, Province of St Francis Xavier: Chronology of Events (2.67A), SSJGB.
41. Various correspondence (PHD 1946/0875, Cons 1003), SROWA.
42. Faulkner, E. to Cook, March 13, 1948 (PHD 1946/0875, Cons 1003), SROWA.
43. Ross, R.A. (Acting Superintendent, Kunmunya Mission) to Cook, June 24, 1948 (PHD 1946/0875, Cons 1003), SROWA.
44. Government files abound with instances of leprosarium abscondments. E.g. eleven incidents in the Northern Territory between 1951 and 1961 are discussed in NAA files E51, 1959/532; F1, 1952/526; F1, 1954/321A; A1658, 258/1/3 and 756/11/7.
45. See for example the regular Sunday exodus to Bagot from East Arm to attend corroborees: Welfare Officer Penhall to Chief Welfare Officer, March 20, 1956 (F1, 1954/321), NAA.
46. E.g. the 1949 Channel Island "walkout." McGlashan, J.G. (Northern Territory Chief Medical Officer) to Metcalfe, A.J. (Commonwealth Director of Health), October 1946 (A1928 715/38/1 Section 3), NAA; Former patient quoted in Hunter, Ernest. 1993. *Aboriginal Health and History: Power and Prejudice in Remote Australia*. Cambridge, New York: Cambridge University Press, 66.
47. 'The Aboriginal Regulations of 1945' (*The Aboriginals Preservation and Protection Act of 1939*, Queensland), 17, 51, 52; 1916 Regulations (*Aborigines Act of 1905*, Western Australia) referred to in Haebich, *For Their Own Good*, 182, 204.
48. Chief Medical Officer (Northern Territory), Draft Memorandum, 181/5, 'Channel Island Leprosarium: The Duties of Superintendent,' October 17, 1949, Daughters of Our Lady of the Sacred Heart Archives, Kensington; 'Leprosarium, Derby, Staff Duties, Superintendent,' May 13, 1954 (Medical Department (MD), 1962/5800, Cons 2506), SROWA.

49. Former patient quoted in Hunter, *Aboriginal Health and History*, 66–67.
50. Nalaielua, Henry (with Sally Jo Bowman). 2006. *No Footprints in the Sand: A Memoir of Kalaupapa*. Honolulu: Watermark Publishing, 78; Anderson, *Colonial Pathologies*, 173, 177.
51. "John" former patient of Fantome Island. Interview with author.
52. Haebich, *For Their Own Good*, 204–205.
53. Director, Queensland Department of Native Affairs (DNA) to Under-Secretary, May 4, 1949 (3A/207, ITM505083), QSA; Former patient cited in Hunter, *Aboriginal Health and History*, 67.
54. Huelin, F. 'Report,' 13 June 13, 1937 (PHD, 1935/0251, Cons 1003), SROWA.
55. St Nérée, Sr to Superintendent, Palm Island, June 19, 1956 (Director of Native Affairs Office, GF/1, Correspondence, Aboriginal and Torres Strait Islander, ID ITM714733), QSA; See Gabriel, Morgan. 'Report on Visit to Fantome Island-April 1953,' 3 (Director of Native Affairs Office, 3A/153, Correspondence, Aboriginal and Torres Strait Islander, ITM505017), QSA, for mention of the Sisters restraining women in the hospital for "immorality."
56. Deputy Director, DNA to Superintendent, Palm Island, September 21, 1951 and Superintendent, Palm Island to Deputy Director, DNA, January 3, 1953, both in (3A/153, ITM50517), QSA.
57. Superintendent, Palm Island to Deputy Director, DNA, January 3, 1953 (3A/153, ITM50517), QSA.
58. Davis, Albert to Atkinson, Everitt, September 20, 1937 (PHD, 1935/0251, Cons 1003), SROWA.
59. Acting Chief Medical Officer (Northern Territory) to Director, Native Affairs Branch, November 17, 1950 (A1928, 715/38/1 Section 1), NAA.
60. Deputy Director of Health (Northern Territory) to Director-General, July 13, 1958 (756/11/3 Section 1), NAA.
61. Julian, Frank to Under-Secretary, February 25, 1944 (DNA Office, 1A/65, PART 1, Correspondence, Aboriginal and Torres Strait Islander, ID ITM501855), QSA. This was a punishment imposed on Palm Island residents. See Finnane, Mark and John McGuire. 2001. 'The Uses of Punishment and Exile: Aborigines in Colonial Australia.' *Punishment and Society* 3, 279, 292–293.
62. Former patient quoted in Hunter, *Aboriginal Health and History*, 66–67.
63. Mother Peter to Bishop Ryan, March 21, 1940 (Box 57, Folder 921), TCA.
64. Former patient quoted in Hunter, *Aboriginal Health and History*, 66–67.
65. Gabriel, Morgan. 'Report on Visit to Fantome Island, April 1953,' 6–7 and Sister St Nérée to Superintendent, Palm Island, June 19, 1956) both at (GF/1, ITM714733), QSA.
66. Cahill, Nida. Letter to unknown recipient. November 15, 1946. MSCD.

67. Derby Leprosarium Regulations, June 2, 1954, WA Health Act, 1911–1953 in *Government Gazette (No. 29)* of 11th June 1954, Section 5 (MD, 1962/5800, Cons 2506), SROWA.
68. Derby Leprosarium Regulations, Section 7.
69. Derby Leprosarium Regulations, Section 8.
70. Humphry, A.H. to Crown Law Officer, Darwin, August 30, 1957 (E51, 1960/277), NAA.
71. Humphry to Henzell, Linley (Western Australia Commissioner of Public Health), April 18, 1957 (MD, 1962/5800, Cons 2506), SROWA.
72. Fryberg, Abraham to Humphry, April 23, 1957 (E51, 1960/277), NAA; Inquest No. 177–1957 (Department of Justice, 176–200, Inquest file, ID ITM349882), QSA.
73. *Register of Heritage Places—Assessment Documentation-Bungarun (Leprosarium), Derby.* February 18, 2000; Henzell to Humphry, April 26, 1957 (MD, 1962/5800, Cons 2506), SROWA.
74. Ibid.; Officer Penhall to Chief Welfare Officer, September 10, 1956 (F1, 1954/321), NAA.
75. Humphry to Crown Law Officer, Darwin, August 30, 1957 (E51, 1960/277), NAA.
76. Leprosarium patient to Director of Health, April 29, 1957 (E51, 1960/277), NAA.
77. Former patients cited in 'Farewell,' *Boab Babbler*, 5 (14), September 1986; former patient quoted in Hunter, *Aboriginal Health and History*, 66; Gibbs, Jack.1995. *Son of Jimmy*. Darwin: Historical Society of the Northern Territory, 117.
78. *Leprosy Ordinance 1954–1957* (NT), Section 31.
79. Acting Chief Medical Officer to Officer Lofthouse, February 5, 1962 and Officer Shaw to Director of Health, February 6, 1962, both in (E51, 1966/732), NAA.
80. Bashford, Alison and Maria Nugent. 2001. 'Leprosy and the Management of Race, Sexuality and Nation in Tropical Australia.' In *Contagion: Historical and Cultural Studies*, ed. Alison Bashford and Claire Hooker. New York and London: Routledge, 109.
81. "Father Nolan" (real name withheld) to Kerrins, Joseph (Provincial Superior, Missionaries of the Sacred Heart, Australia), October 12, 1946 (Prov. Corr., N.T.Darwin, 1946), MSCK.
82. 'Reports and recommendations resulting from inquiry held at Channel Island,' October 1946, and McGlashan to Metcalfe, October 22, 1946, both in (A1928, 715/38/1 Section 30), NAA.
83. Gribble, E.R. to Archdeacon, October 26, 1949 (Australian Board of Missions, Further Records 1873–1978, MLMSS 4503 Add On 1822, Box 10 (69), G9), Mitchell Library, Sydney.

84. Cahill, Nita to Minister for Health, July 1, 1948 (A1658, 756/11/7), NAA.
85. McKenna, Nick to Kerrins, December 3, 1946 (Prov. Corr., N.T.Darwin, 1946), MSCK.
86. Cook to Metcalfe, March 30, 1949 (A1658, 756/11/7), NAA.
87. Fantome Island patient to Secretary, Relatives and Friends Association, August 25, 1952 (ITM505017), QSA.
88. Ibid.
89. Ibid.
90. Deputy Director DNA to Superintendent, Palm Island, November 22, 1951 (ITM505017), QSA.
91. Superintendent, Palm Island to Deputy Director, DNA, September 17, 1951 (ITM505017), QSA.
92. St. Nérée, Sr to Superintendent, Palm Island, September 2, 1951 (ITM505017), QSA.
93. Various documents in (A1928, 715/38/1 Section 3), NAA.

CHAPTER 8

Missionary Men and the Indigenous Leprosaria 1940–c.1955

Government engagement of Catholic Sisters at the leprosaria was viewed as advantageous by sections of the Australian Catholic Church, as it opened a new mission field in which priests and Brothers would naturally take part. Senior clerics, having been instrumental in brokering the Sisters' appointments in the 1930s and early-1940s, continued close involvement with the institutions, drawing them into the small but expanding network of mission stations and schools under their domain in the north and north-west. This chapter examines how the Catholic Church pursued its missionary ends in the leprosarium through the work of its male religious in their roles as chaplains and superintendents in the 1940s and early-1950s. The focus is on Channel and Fantome Islands, where isolation lessened the gaze of rival denominations caught up in the prevalent sectarianism between Protestants and Catholics. For many individual Australian Catholic priests and Brothers, as with the Sisters, the leprosy apostolate was a long-held aspiration and a meaningful way to "spend themselves in the salvation of souls" in emulation of legendary religious figures, such as Damien of Molokai.[1] But, under female authority and far from their religious communities, the leprosaria, for several men, fell far short of such promises.

C. Robson, *Missionary Women, Leprosy and Indigenous Australians, 1936–1986*, https://doi.org/10.1007/978-3-031-05796-0_8

The Catholic Male Missionary Impulse

Among the first Catholic chaplains to the Sisters were William Henschke and Patrick Moloney, priests of the Missionaries of the Sacred Heart (MSC) order. They arrived in the early 1940s at Channel and Fantome Islands, respectively, where, according to reports, few patients were of the Catholic faith.[2] Their experiences as missionaries and the attitudes they developed in regard to Indigenous people informed the way they went about the evangelisation of leprosarium patients. Aged sixty-four and fifty-four, respectively, Moloney and Henschke had put the most active phases of their religious vocations behind them when they began their leprosarium ministries, yet they both remained highly driven missionaries. Henschke was a veteran of Indigenous missionary work, having spent many years at the side of Bishop Gsell on Bathurst Island Mission, before heading up the Darwin parish.[3] His efforts to have the SSJG Sisters installed at Channel Island and his subsequent involvement in the appointment of the DOLSH Sisters have been discussed in Chapter 4. Moloney was known for his pioneering endeavours at Palm Island, Alice Springs and Menindee in the 1930s and had been a main protagonist of the Church's interwar remote mission enterprise, as has also been briefly discussed. For Moloney, Indigenous missionary work was part of a collective moral duty, specifically directed towards addressing the wrongs inflicted by unscrupulous white Australians.[4] His letter to a government minister in 1938 to protest moves to close his Alice Springs mission station couches this duty in explicitly political terms, while it demonstrates his contempt for claims of Australian egalitarianism:

> We boast of our civilisation, our culture and advancement, our broad-mindedness and willingness to give everyone a fair deal, yet we have shot, poisoned and starved to almost complete extinction a most noble black race. The soil of this Continent has been steeped in black blood, and anyone who takes up the cause of the few that remain, becomes as bitterly hated even as are the blacks.[5]

There seemed to be no doubt in the minds of Henschke and Moloney that amends to the Indigenous could be made, in the words of their associate, Reverend Johnston, "by putting within their reach the Faith and all its blessings."[6] Under state health detention laws, the leprosarium ensured the men had a captive population—Indigenous people, who in other circumstances, might reject or never experience the overtures of missionaries. As one priest noted of the Derby leprosarium, "Avenues of approach to the pagans closed to the missionaries through bigotry or difficulty of access are now being opened up in this perhaps providential manner."[7]

Moloney and Henschke displayed a self-assurance in their methods that contrasted with the Sisters' approach to evangelising the patients. Despite being allowed only as visitors, both men slipped unobtrusively into full-time residence on the islands, taking up makeshift accommodation, and boldly flouting the health regulations that kept most other people away. Clergy of other denominations were given only visiting permits and, with access to the island difficult, they could not possibly attain the dominant presence the Catholic priests achieved. The men were both known for their engaging personalities and friendly paternal ways. Henschke is remembered as "a gentle giant" who, on returning to Channel Island from a trip to town, brought with him a huge bag containing chewing gum for the children and tobacco for the adults. The patients, especially the women, would gather around him to hear him tell stories.[8] Converting an old building into a chapel specifically for them, he hoped to "gradually make an impression on the patients."[9]

Moloney and Henschke, as with several other priests, performed numerous baptisms at the leprosaria, most without full instruction of the patients or their acceptance Catholicisim.[10] In this practice, they differed from other MSC mission veterans such as Bishop F.X. Gsell who held little concern for the prospect of eternal damnation for the unconverted.[11] Yet, perhaps in the leprosarium of the 1940s, when the death toll was high, there was more urgency to ensure patients could die as Catholics, so that "our poor Australian brothers obtain [their] real inheritance," as one priest expressed it.[12] Success was measured in numbers baptised and confirmed, in Catholic weddings, and head counts in church. In 1954, resident priest, Fr Monckton, could report of the Fantome Island Leprosarium in the *Townsville Catholic News*,

> Since the Mission was established, there have been eighty-two baptisms, forty-three confirmations and thirty-eight burials. The total number buried on Fantome is eighty-two so nearly half of those who died was won to the faith... there were ten Catholic marriages in total.[13]

Proselytisation, if attempted by the Sisters, seemed to have occurred with caution, whereas the priests confidently and quite openly tried to bring all they could to their Church without any concern for existing religious beliefs. One case at Fantome Island suggests that the priests' evangelical fervour left very little space for the supposedly multi-denominational nature of the institution. In 1942, Moloney administered Baptism and first Holy Communion to a young girl who "belonged" to the Church of England, without the consent of her legal guardian.[14] The outrage of Palm Island Anglican minister, E.R. Gribble, and his resultant campaign to discredit the Sisters in the eyes of the public, led Mother Peter to ask Moloney to allow the girl to return to her former Church which he refused to do.[15] The girl fled into the bush every Sunday, no doubt preferring to avoid Mass altogether rather than be caught up in this clerics' tug-of-war.[16] Mother Peter, apart from her upset at the resultant publicity, regretted the damage it caused to the Sisters' relations with the Anglicans, telling Moloney, "If we acted squarely with Canon Gribble he would act squarely with us…He passes by our very door and never calls in through you."[17] Yet, for Moloney, the patients owed the Church their allegiance as gratitude to the Sisters. He was critical of a Baptist patient who, on her deathbed, refused one Sister's attempts to baptise her as a Catholic, as the former "not only nursed her, but taught her in school."[18]

From the late 1940s, the Fantome Island 'Catholic mission' surged forward. Having completed the building of a church and presbytery, the MSCs withdrew, due to a shortage of priests, and Bishop Ryan took the project in hand, appointing Father Basil Foster, a diocesan priest, as resident chaplain in 1947, and paying him £100 annual stipend.[19] Fantome Island was the only leprosarium to retain a Catholic priest in formal full-time residence, a position that continued almost until its closure in 1973. More than any other religious, Foster worked to transform the leprosarium into a Catholic mission. He made converts, both of the living and dying, with vigour. He also spent much time in giving patients religious instruction and, to this end, published a small periodical, the *Catholic Koro*, written "in simple language which would confine itself to stating plainly the doctrines of the Catholic faith" (Fig. 8.1).[20]

Foster also turned his energies to the visual and the ceremonial aspects of the practice of the Catholic faith. The ubiquitous religious statuary and the elaborate vestments that typically define a site of Catholic worship first found their place in a government leprosarium under his influence. Overlooking one beach, a statue of Mary Immaculate "high on a column of gleaming white…proclaims the faith and love of the children of Fantome Island" while Our Lady of Lourdes, illuminated at night by

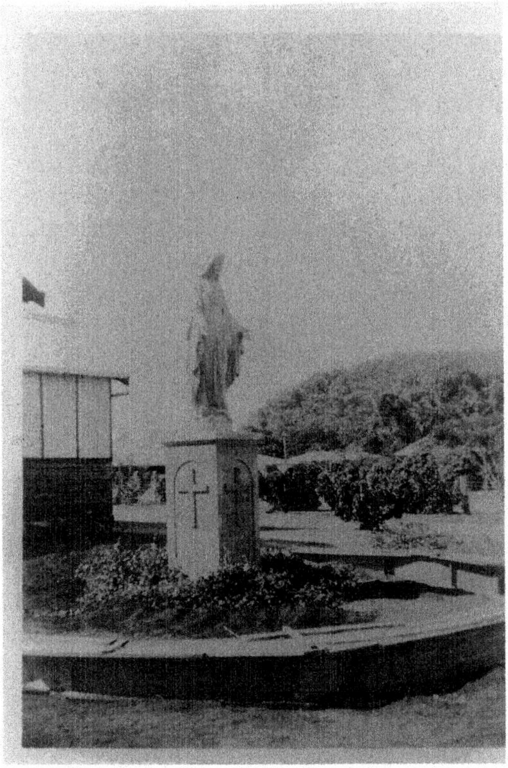

Fig. 8.1 Statue of Mary at Fantome Island (James Cook University Library Special Collections)

electric light, looked from her grotto.[21] Together they were reminiscent of the Marian spirit alive in the Catholic world outside, emblematic of a common struggle against "immorality, communism and war."[22] Foster added a "wooded grove with outdoor Stations of the Cross and shrines of some saints."[23] He began the tradition of holding Eucharistic processions on the island each year on the feast day of Corpus Christi, as celebrated in Australia's cities.[24]

Sacred objects were not merely ornaments or even devices to assist the religious staff in their spiritual reflections. They were markers of Catholic territory, etched into the virgin landscape as statues, or shifting through it as the flowing habits of the religious, impervious to the rusted ideals and dented hopes of the succession of missionaries who bent their heads beneath them. They suggested, if not the victory of a sturdy Catholic patient congregation, then at least an assertion that this should be so, a prospect that filled some on the other side of the sectarian divide with a fear for the spiritual fate of the patients under their own ministries.

The mission-building occurring at Fantome Island was not implemented to the same extent on Channel Island. The Catholic missionaries, throughout the years 1945–1950 saved their plans for the proposed relocation of the leprosarium to Melville Island where the MSCs already operated a mission for mixed race children. Here, Henschke hoped, would be "a wonderful opportunity to care for and nurse poor afflicted people and to do good for their souls whereas little can be done in the present place as other denominations interfere."[25] But reports concluded that Melville Island had all the deficiencies of the current leprosarium site, being even more remote from services and lacking the water supply needed for subsistence farming. The consequences of its proximity to the mission on Bathurst Island, for example, mixing between the mission residents and the leprosarium patients, were also of concern.[26] Fantome Island also suffered the disadvantages of distance from services and lack of water but the leprosarium remained there and isolation served the Catholic mission project well. In 1950, recently appointed bishop of Darwin, John O'Loughlin, overturned the plans for Melville Island on the abovementioned grounds, stating that a mainland site close to Darwin should be chosen, despite the government's offer of the entire management of the new leprosarium to the MSCs.[27] His decision was evidence of a change of guard in the Catholic missionary hierarchy in which practical and materially beneficial considerations outweighed uncompromised missionary zeal.

At the Derby leprosarium, government warnings against the overt proselytisation of patients meant that the evangelisation of patients was attempted in subtle ways. In 1947, the Pallottine Fathers established a parish centre in the town of Derby, bringing priests, for the first time, a short drive away from the leprosarium. Many patients at Derby had no prior Christian affiliations so conversion entailed the introduction of entirely new beliefs. Former visiting priest from the 1950s, Fr Joe

Kearney explained that most religious instruction at Derby was provided by catechists who were also patients. Each Saturday, he would offer encouragement while the male catechist instructed male patients. Corresponding arrangements were organised for the female patients under the supervision of one of the Sisters. Instruction continued for about six months before a person was ready for baptism. Fr Kearney has pointed out that having learned the Christian message from other Indigenous, rather than from Europeans, patients became motivated to pass on their new beliefs to others in their communities after leaving the leprosarium.[28]

But Catholicism did not have a monopoly on these activities, according to Kearney, who remembered that Protestant patients also instructed others in the ways of their faith.[29] Rather than dictate the direction of Christianity at Derby, there is evidence that visits of the Catholic priests spurred ministers of other denominations into acting to ensure their Churches were represented in the leprosarium and that patients from their missions did not transfer their affiliation to Catholicism.[30] They became regular visitors, presiding over services in a second church built for use by all Christians other than Catholics. New patients joined cliques identified by a common home region, at least several of which assumed a particular Christian affiliation and practised their religion under the guidance of a senior member, thus strengthening the multi-denominational character of the leprosarium.

These practices also occurred at the other two leprosaria but were not so successful in competing with the dominance of Catholicism. However, with the Darwin leprosarium's relocation to the mainland in 1955, Methodist and Anglican ministers could more readily access patients who had originated from missions under their societies' control, holding separate services each Sunday. Being drawn to the festivity and music of Mass, some patients reportedly attended every service, regardless of the faith they identified with.[31] Catholic male religious, therefore, played significant roles both in their direct evangelisation of patients into their Church and by inadvertently providing the stimulus for missionaries of other Churches to do the same, with the result that, generally, Christian worship and the promotion of Christian beliefs proliferated in the leprosaria. This phenomenon has been noted also by historian Noel Loos who argues that United Aborigines Mission and Anglican missionaries tolerated one another's activities on Palm and Fantome Islands until the arrival of Catholic religious, and, then, "Never had black souls seemed so precious."[32] It also goes some way to explaining why not all patients who first found Christianity in leprosaria, later identified with Catholicism.[33]

Martyrdom and Missionary Men

Throughout the 1940s and beyond, missionary societies and the Catholic press continued to affirm the sanctity of the relationship between leprosy patient and missionary, emphasising the spiritual richness of the Australian leprosarium ministry. Published articles spoke of Christ's presence or another Damien of Molokai in the person of the religious, sometimes articulating the great sacrifices they made.[34] Several were written by visiting priests on short stopovers as they toured the missions. They wrote rapturously of the devout and appreciative 'native leper,' transformed from "roam[ing] the bush with his tribe in pain and misery" to "finding peace of mind and joy of soul" under the care of the religious.[35] The impression was invariably given of a flourishing Catholic community who "flocked to the Communion rails in heart-warming numbers."[36] The administration of the sacraments, in which the priest shares a more intimate interaction with the recipient, was conveyed with disquieting drama and pathos, the patients' disabilities juxtaposed against their pious humility:

> That night I heard the Confessions of the Catholic lepers. Again I nearly cried with sadness as the poor creatures humbly murmured their peccadilloes in the rasping voices produced by the disease...[37]

Another priest, writing of Palm Sunday rituals, mused, "It was touching to see the lepers reverently kiss the palm and receive them, sometimes with fingerless hands."[38] And another explained how the prayer [of communion] "is said with deeper meaning by a priest when he distributes Communion to the sick – particularly to those afflicted with leprosy."[39]

Some Australian priests and brothers expressed particular interest in working with leprosy patients. Of the Channel Island ministry, Fr Henschke had written "it was the ambition of my life realised," and for Brother "Lucas", the superintendent's job was "special work" and had been his "ambition for years."[40] Before accepting an appointment at Fantome Island in 1954, Father Roch Allen OFM, had "been begging for years for missionary work among the lepers."[41] Father Aquinas Howard

OFM, who missed out on the position, was, according to another religious, "very anxious to devote his life to the lepers."[42] There was competition for leprosarium work between men of the same order, of different Catholic orders, and of different Christian denominations. It was highly sought, both as a church missionary project and as a personal religious endeavour.

The misty ambitions of would-be Damiens and the biblical rhetoric of passing priests, however, did not necessarily reflect the reality that many male missionaries faced in their positions as leprosarium personnel. Mission warhorses, Moloney, and Henschke, survived by their indomitable optimism and on the strength of their old rock-solid vocations. But for the young and more vulnerable who'd joined "the army of the real heroes of the world in the ceaseless search for souls," postings at the leprosarium often descended into disappointment, anguish, and, not uncommonly, injury to physical and mental health. The real sacrifices they faced were not the risk of contracting the disease or sharing life with those "selected to undergo Purgatory on earth"; they were the attendant solitude, the isolation and feelings of powerlessness.[43]

Provincial superiors did not delegate their most promising or capable missionaries to permanent positions at the leprosaria, being alive to the shortcomings of the Australian leprosaria as mission projects from an early date. In 1941, just a year after the Fantome Island leprosarium opened, the MSC Provincial Superior, Father Kerrins, and the Bishop Ryan of Townsville agreed that the "elderly man or the man with a hobby is the type of chaplain required."[44] In 1945, the former was thinking of "some old mission priest who may be happy to spend his days attending to the lepers."[45] More active and skilled missionaries were preferred for building and maintaining large mission stations overseas or on the small Indigenous stations where talents in carpentry, mechanics and agriculture were necessary.[46] The evangelisation of thousands of Papuans took priority to fifty Indigenous Australians when personnel were scarce. Often, however, short-term or intermittent postings of men of a variety of ages and temperaments were made to the leprosaria, stretching out to many months or years.

The priests who served at Fantome Island in the early-1940s found the leprosarium was not the missionary enterprise they envisaged. There were never more than seventy-five patients in residence and admissions hardly kept up with the numbers who died. Many were either firm adherents of other churches, or the old, frail and dying, leaving little for the priests to do apart from conducting a disproportionate number of deathbed baptisms, leading one priest to comment on learning of his departure from the island, "I am delighted to be able to do something besides sit down and watch lepers get daily worse."[47] Church congregations were very small and individuals found to have little understanding of the faith, due to hasty conversions by over-enthusiastic predecessors.[48] Fr "Giles" found himself overcome by inertia when it came to extending himself from chaplaincy to evangelistic work. The prevalence of "paganism"

> ...one might imagine would stir a zealous man to vigorous action. Yes! Sitting in the front seat of the chapel it might and does, but when one comes bump up against it all, it staggers one, gives a jolt and you hear yourself saying, 'Cui bono?' They're doing alright! Why worry? Say daily mass for the Sisters, say your office...[49]

In the eyes of several of these young ambitious priests, Fantome Island compared unfavourably with the overseas missions run by the MSCs such as New Guinea, China, and the Pacific islands. Fr "Murphy" was disappointed to hear he was not to be transferred away as he had been "dreaming of New Guinea."[50] Fr "Biggins" rejoiced in his own transfer there.[51] Such missions boasted thousands of potential converts, unspoiled by rival Christian denominations, and the 'natives' were reputedly far more amenable to evangelisation than Indigenous Australians.[52] These then were the places where a missionary could feel he was doing worthwhile work.

Several male missionaries found the spiritual and intellectual separation from their fellow religious at the leprosarium extremely challenging, leading some to the collapse of their mental or physical health. Whereas the leprosarium Sisters, once established, formed communities of at least four women, the priests and brothers lived mostly well away from the company of their confreres. For young priests, turned out of twentieth-century seminaries, where for many years they had learnt and lived in a communal environment of likeminded religious, the leprosarium was a lonely experience. Priests who took up work in suburban parishes, in contrast, "shared experiences, exchanged ideas and told each other about the books and articles they were reading."[53] Fr Giles found small talk with the Fantome Islanders poor compensation. "After all they have never done 'Three years' nor are particularly interested in Plain Chant!"[54]

For missionary priests, work as the Sisters' chaplains was sometimes unrewarding and it distracted from their main vocational purpose. As a 1953 authority on the subject explained, the chaplain's role was very different to the usual ministries of the priest as it was not "a question of doing good, spreading the kingdom of God and procuring the salvation of souls," but centred on perfecting a community of "chosen souls."[55] The MSC fathers at Fantome Island found the Sisters overly demanding in their continual requests for more frequent Mass while simultaneously running the Palm Island mission. They also resented what they saw as unwarranted intervention by the Sisters in their attempts to fulfil their missionary projects. Fr Moloney objected to Mother Peter's criticism of his proselytisation of the patients, telling his superior, "Mother Peter was parish priest before I came and she can't get used to the change over," and, mimicking her, "'Who are you?- you are only the chaplain.'"[56] In a sense, the roles of Sister and priest had been reversed, the latter losing the seniority and centrality he'd come to expect on the mission station or in the parish, and, the former, the linchpin upon which hinged the Catholic mission imperative at the leprosarium.

The Franciscan Missionaries of Mary who replaced the Our Lady Help of Christians Sisters in 1944 continued to voice complaints about the chaplaincy work of the MSCs and, after their departure in 1947, of Father Foster. When their longstanding request for a resident priest of their co-fraternity, the Order of Friars Minor, was eventually satisfied in 1952, relations appeared to improve, or, perhaps any friction was kept more carefully under wraps.

Between 1943 and 1955, a series of MSC Brothers filled the role of government superintendent at Channel Island, apart from a short interlude in the late-1940s. The Northern Territory administration was particularly grateful for the services of Denis McCarthy, the first Brother superintendent, who arrived during the Darwin military occupation when most laymen had been evacuated. Experience on Indigenous Catholic missions was qualification enough for the work brief, listed as ordering and distributing all supplies and rations, and controlling visitor permits.[57] Only later did it become clear that other, more demanding duties were expected, including looking after machinery, organising male patient labour, and maintaining law and order.[58] McCarthy's labour came cheaply as, for the five years he held this position, neither he nor his religious society received any financial remuneration from the government, not even the small sum paid to the Sisters per week for their personal requirements.[59] Nor was McCarthy, as a religious Brother, likely to ask for better conditions either for himself or for the others on the island. Whereas for the Sisters, a certain—albeit poor—standard of accommodation was always provided, McCarthy moved into a garage, open at both ends. A feature on Channel Island in his order's journal, *The Annals*, portrayed him as a willing martyr living in a "tin shed," but he "did not come here for a holiday, he would tell you, so he does not want a mansion. He ought to be satisfied."[60]

McCarthy, who "likes doing little pottering jobs about the place, is easy tempered, and religious," was soon noted by his colleagues to be neither adept at either carrying out repairs nor at evangelising the patients.[61] His superiors were not worried, deciding his talents lay elsewhere and "he will do with his prayers what many others could not do with their efficiency."[62] It became clear, however, that it was more his despondency than lack of skill that led to such reticence. Within the year, he asked for a transfer back to the missions where he could avail daily Mass.[63] However, over the next five years, repeated requests and declining spirits were all met with refusal by his superiors to authorise his removal, as no replacement could be found. The Brothers who had expressed interest were either deemed completely unsuitable or were needed for their skills on the missions.

McCarthy's actions continued to prove to his fellow religious and his superiors that he was unfit to perform the work. Father "Murphy" noted that he tried to do the work of three men without ever requesting additional assistance and that "for weeks he has been tinkering with the fridge engine instead of reporting its failure…I won't be surprised if the next issue of the *Darwin Standard* has glaring headlines, 'No refrigeration at lep.'"[64] After a group of patients walked off the island in 1946 to protest at conditions, a government inquiry revealed him to be ineffectual at enforcing the sexual segregation policy and maintaining the orderly behaviour of the patients.[65] But the accompanying recommendation that he be replaced with a layman was not at this time enacted.

Several MSC priests protested the injustice of leaving McCarthy to endure appalling living conditions and an onerous workload, and pushed to have their Brothers permanently withdrawn from the superintendent's position. The current Local Superior found nothing noble in a martyrdom arising from government thrift, unlike his predecessor, Henschke. In 1948, a similarly disapproving "Murphy" argued that "I do not think our Constitution or Statutes can justify his presence there."[66] The current documents stressed that MSC mission work was to be voluntary and, furthermore, that "missionaries be so placed on mission stations that no one suffers spiritual harm because of isolation."[67] It was only in 1949, after religious nursing staff on Channel Island were implicated in charges of neglect towards a dying patient (but were subsequently exonerated) that Bishop Gsell finally agreed to withdraw McCarthy. He and other senior clergy believed the charges were part of a communist plot to remove the Catholic religious from the leprosarium and did not want the MSCs subjected to further attack.[68]

That the MSC superiors prevaricated for so long before authorising McCarthy's removal suggests that his importance for them lay not in how he performed his role as superintendent, or even as a religious, but in the mere fact that he, as a Catholic missionary, continued to occupy the position. Throughout discussions around his removal, the superiors had always expressed concerns about the consequences for their missionary ambitions at the leprosarium if, in the likely event they could not replace him, the position was vacated. A lay superintendent in his place, some thought, would make the Sisters so uncomfortable, they would resign their positions, and, if a Communist sympathiser, would influence the patients with his beliefs.[69] Even more worrying was the possibility that a Protestant missionary might take the job. Bishop Gsell believed "the Protestants are looking for the place. They'll jump in as soon as we leave. It would be a disgrace to our church and society."[70] Even if the resident Catholic male religious was not effective in making mission inroads at the leprosarium, his presence at least prevented any other denominations from doing the same.

As government authorities quickly discovered, a religious Brother as superintendent was their best asset in masking the appalling conditions at the leprosarium. The layman installed after McCarthy's departure in 1949 lasted just nine months, resigning after alerting the newspapers to the severe water shortage on the island.[71] These were old problems, known to government officials, but, since the 1930s, they had decided not to make any improvements pending the relocation of the leprosarium to a new site. After the MSCs agreed to supply another Brother on condition that more comfortable quarters and financial remuneration be supplied, things settled back almost to the same quiet privations of the previous years. Brother Lilwall "attends to the welfare of some 200 leper patients. He is often required to act as peacemaker amongst the natives, maintain the various buildings, supervise the work of natives who are capable of working and a multitude of other duties...his day begins at 4 am and he is often still working at 11 pm."[72] Notably, by minimising outside influences, his presence protected the interests of both his Church and the government, allowing them to continue operations as they intended. Although he had a "grueling time," he held out until 1956, just after the leprosarium was re-established on the mainland, spelling the end to its insularity and demanding a larger and more complex administrative staff structure than any religious order could supply. The Director-General of Health "regret[ted] that he leaves us at a time when I feel the road was becoming a little easier."[73]

* * *

Whereas Catholic nursing Sisters mostly evangelised their patients discreetly, the priests used ceremony, sacraments and the church to "dazzle the natives with mitre and crozier."[74] Some, in addition, brought imposing, charismatic personalities and gifts. Familiarisation with the non-Catholic patients had to be cultivated in an obvious and self-conscious way, unlike the bonds that formed more easily in the nursing and educational activities undertaken by the Sisters. The Catholic priests showed no hesitation in their determination to bring both the dying and living, whether "pagan" or Protestant, to what they believed to be the true Church, fuelling and fearing the sectarian competition in their midst. Male missionaries of other Churches responded by intensifying their efforts to claim the souls of the patients, resulting in a powerful yet diverse Christianising impulse, wherever the conditions allowed for their influence to be felt.

Yet, as this study shows, leprosarium work in Australia largely failed to fulfil the expectations of the male religious. Its isolation, the thin harvest of souls, the limitations of the men's official roles as chaplain and superintendent, and clashes with the religious Sisters put this apostolate, as one Catholic magazine phrased it, "on the margin of mission life."[75] Loneliness, boredom and disempowerment at times saw a lifelong commitment to the 'lepers' commuted to a short and unhappy sojourn.

Despite low numbers of converts and disenchanted missionaries, the Catholic Church continued for longer than was justifiable to use male religious to maintain a dominant presence in the leprosaria. Of paramount importance for the Church was to always be able to claim that the leprosarium was a Catholic mission. By the middle of the 1950s, the influence of the Catholic male missionaries in the leprosaria had waned. In the Northern Territory, Bishop O'Loughlin's decision to turn down the government's offer of the leprosarium on Melville Island, and his withdrawal of the Brothers as superintendents, implied different priorities in which the men under his authority were not to be martyrs for the government, no matter how attractive spiritually the leprosy apostolate might appear. On Fantome Island, as will be explained, there were no more than about twenty-six patients after 1955, so at this leprosarium, too, the Catholic mission project lulled. Visiting Catholic priests continued to provide pastoral care to leprosarium patients at East Arm and Derby but, as time went on, they increasingly made way for missionaries of other denominations.

Notes

1. Missionaries of the Sacred Heart (MSC). 1942. *Constitution of the Society of Missionaries of the Sacred Heart of Jesus*. Kensington: Sacred Heart Monastery, no. 3.
2. Henschke, William to Kerrins, Joseph (MSC Provincial Superior), December 2, 1943 (Provincial Correspondence N.T. Darwin, 1943), MSC Archives Kensington (MSCK); Father "Biggins" (name withheld) to Kerrins, August 25, 1941 (Palm Island 1940–1941), MSCK.
3. Littleton, James J. ed. 1992. *Brotherhood in Mission: Deceased Missionaries of the Sacred Heart, Australia 1882–1991*. Coogee: MSC Provincial House, 75.
4. See Chapter 2 for discussion of the Catholic Indigenous mission endeavour in the 1930s as a national duty.
5. Moloney, Fr P.J. to Blain, Macalister A., January 3, 1938 (A1, 1938/403), National Archives of Australia (NAA).
6. Johnston, H. 1936. 'Australian Catholics and the Aboriginals.' In *The National Eucharistic Congress Melbourne, Australia, December 2nd–9th, 1934*, ed. J.M. Murphy and F. Moynihan. Melbourne: Advocate Press, 177.
7. Breslin, D. 'Aussie Nuns and Aussie Lepers.' *Catholic Missions*, March 1947, 14.
8. "Sr Jeanne" OLSH (name withheld). Interview with author. Typed transcript. Recorded at Kensington, New South Wales, August 18, 2008.
9. Henschke to Kerrins, December 2, 1943 (Prov. Corr., N.T. Darwin 1943), MSCK; Palm Island and Fantome Island Catholic Register, Townsville Cathedral Archives (TCA).

10. Henschke to Kerrins, January 8, 1944 (Prov. Corr., N.T. Darwin 1944), MSCK.
11. Hearn, Peter. 2003. *A Theology of Mission: An Analysis of the Theology of Mission of the Catholic Diocese of Darwin in Its Ministry to Aboriginal People During the Episcopy of John O'Loughlin MSC 1949–85*. Kensington: Nelen Yubu Missiological Unit, 30–31.
12. Fantome Island priest (name withheld) to Kerrins, August 25, 1941 (Palm Island 1940–1941), MSCK.
13. Monckton, Fr V. 1954. 'Fantome Island: Our Diocesan Leper Station.' *Townsville Catholic News (TCN),* December 1, 11.
14. Moloney to Kerrins, November 7, 1942 (Palm Island 1942–1943), MSCK; Mother Peter to Bishop Ryan, November 10, 1942 (1145, Box 57, Folder 921), TCA.
15. Moloney to Kerrins, November 12, 1942 (Palm Island 1942–1943), MSCK. Claims in Queensland Protestant periodical, the *Clarion*, of October 1942, that the Fantome Island Sisters were forcing their patients to attend Catholic church services probably originated in this incident. The Health Department asked for a written response from Mother Peter. See Acting Secretary, Dept of Public Health (Queensland) to Mother Peter, November 2, 1942, and her reply of November 9, 1942 (1145, Box 57, Folder 921), TCA.
16. Mother Peter to Ryan, Bishop Hugh, November 10, 1942 (1145, Box 57, Folder 921), TCA; Moloney to Kerrins, November 7, 1942 (Palm Island 1942–1943), MSCK.
17. Moloney to Kerrins, November 7, 1942 (Palm Island 1942–1943), MSCK.
18. Ibid.
19. Diocesan Secretary to Foster, Fr Basil, September 9, 1948 (Holdings, Box 108, Folder 1), TCA.
20. Foster to Ryan, May 15, 1954 (1140, Box 56, Folder 916), TCA.
21. Monckton, V. 1957. 'Fantome Island: Our Diocesan Leper Station.' TCN, December 1, 10; Monckton, V. 1957. 'A Visit to Fantome and Palm Islands.' *TCN*, June 1, 9.
22. Massam, Katharine. 1996. *Sacred Threads: Catholic Spirituality in Australia 1922–1962*. Sydney: University of New South Wales Press, 92.
23. Monckton, 'Fantome Island,' 11; Ryan to Foster, July 11, 1952 (1141, Box 56, Folder 917), TCA.
24. Allen, Fr Roch. 1962. 'Eucharistic Devotion on Fantome Island Leprosarium.' *TCN,* August 1, 4.
25. Henschke to Kerrins, March 29, 1945 (Prov. Corr., N.T. Darwin 1943), MSCK.
26. O'Loughlin, Bishop John and Humphry, A.H., 'Report of a Visit to Proposed Site on Melville,' June 22, 1950 (A1658, 756/10/3), NAA.

27. O'Loughlin to Barbour, C.S. (Chief Medical Officer), July 10, 1950 (A1658, 756/10/3), NAA.
28. Kearney, Father Joseph SAC. Interview with author, Pallottine Rossmoyne Community, Western Australia, October 5, 2009.
29. Ibid.
30. Secretary of Correspondence, United Aborigines Mission to Atkinson, Everitt (Western Australia Commissioner of Public Health), July 17, 1937 (Public Health Department (PHD), 1935/0251, Cons 1003), State Records Office Western Australia (SROWA).
31. Whelan, Sister Marion OLSH. Interview with author. Typed transcript. Recorded at Kensington, New South Wales, August 12, 2008; Carroll, Sister Benedicta OLSH. Interview with author. Typed transcript. Recorded at Kensington, New South Wales, September 9, 2008.
32. Loos, Noel. 2007. *White Christ, Black Cross: The Emergence of a Black Church*. Australian Capital Territory: Aboriginal Studies Press, 82.
33. Bedford, Paddy. 1997. 'God Knows.' In *The Telling of Stories: A Spiritual Journey of Kimberley Aboriginal People*, ed. Peter Bibby. Western Australia: Catholic Education Office, Kimberley Region, 37; Charles Darwin University, 'Gawirrin Gumana—Biography,' http://www.cdu.edu.au/newsroom/documents/biography-gawirrin-gumana.pdf. Accessed 27 June 2011.
34. Morris, H.D. 1952. 'Darwin and Channel Island.' *The Annals of Our Lady of the Sacred Heart (The Annals)*, October 1, 228–229; Foley, Frederic. 1955. 'Leper Christmas.' *Messenger*, January 1, 32; 'Chaplain for Leprosarium.' *TCN*, February 1, 1947, 3; '"Ad Multos Annos:" Two Priestly Jubilarians.' TCN, January 1, 1953, 4; Monckton, 'Fantome Island,' 10; Monckton, 'A Visit to Fantome and Palm Islands,' 9; Eldridge, John. 1942. 'An Island Lazaret: The Story of an Heroic Missionary Enterprise.' *The Annals*, February 2, 41.
35. Morris, 'Darwin and Channel Island,' 229.
36. Whitty, Thomas. 1948. 'The Lepers' Faith.' *The Annals*, July 1, 212; see also Foley, 'Leper Christmas,' 32.
37. Morris, 'Darwin and Channel Island,' 229.
38. Whitty, 'The Lepers' Faith,' 212.
39. Copas, V.P. 1957. 'Lepers in North Australia.' *The Annals,* June 1, 1957, 168.
40. Brother "Lucas" (name withheld) to Kerrins, March 31, 1943, and Henschke to Kerrins, April 29, 1943, both in (Prov. Corr., N.T. Darwin 1943), MSCK.
41. Gleeson, Joseph to Ryan, February 9, 1954 (1140, Box 56, Folder 916), TCA.
42. Ibid.; de la Merci, Sister Maree to Ryan, October 2, 1946 (1140, Box 56, Folder 916), TCA.

43. '"Unclean, Unclean!" The Lepers: August Missionary Intention.' *Catholic Missions*, August 1, 1935, 3.
44. Kerrins to Ryan, November 18, 1941 (Palm Island 1943–1947), MSCK.
45. Kerrins to Fr "Giles" (name withheld), August 27, 1945 (Palm Island 1944–1946), MSCK.
46. Gsell, Bishop F.X. to Breene, Aidan (MSC Provincial Superior), August 21, 1948 (Prov. Corr., N.T. Darwin 1948), MSCK; Father "Murphy" (name withheld) to Breene, August 18, 1950 (Prov. Corr., N.T. Darwin 1950), MSCK.
47. Father "Biggins" (name withheld) to Kerrins, December 4, 1940 (Palm Island 1940–1941), MSCK.
48. Father "Giles" to Kerrins, June 22, 1942 (Palm Island 1944–1946), MSCK.
49. Father "Giles" to Kerrins, ~ 1946 (Palm Island 1944–1946), MSCK.
50. Father "Murphy" to Kerrins, December 17, 1944 (Palm Island 1943–1947), MSCK.
51. Fr "Biggins" to Kerrins, December 4, 1940 (Palm Island 1940–1941), MSCK.
52. For example, in 1943, 45 priests and 15 brothers of the MSC served 124,000 Catholics in the Philippines diocese of Surigao; 64 priests and 50 brothers served at the MSC mission at Rabaul where there were 64,000 Catholics (*The Annals*, October 1, 1943, 184).
53. Campion, Edmund. 2009. *Ted Kennedy: Priest of Redfern*. Kew East: David Lovell Publishing, 28.
54. Father "Giles" to Kerrins, c. 1942 (Palm Island 1944–1946), MSCK.
55. le Terrier, Canon. 1956. 'The Chaplain.' In *The Direction of Nuns*. Trans. Lancelot C. Shepherd. London: Blackfriars Publications, 123.
56. Moloney to Kerrins, November 7, 1942 (Palm Island 1942–1943), MSCK.
57. McCarthy, Brother Denis to Kerrins, September 28, 1943 (Prov. Corr., N.T. Darwin 1943), MSCK.
58. Commonwealth of Australia, Department of Health, Northern Territory Division, 'Channel Island Leper Hospital—Organisation,' May 6, 1946, Daughters of Our Lady of the Sacred Heart Archives, Kensington, New South Wales.
59. In 1949, after McCarthy left Channel Island, the MSC received £1000 from the Commonwealth Health Department to cover the three years since control of the leprosarium passed to the Northern Territory Medical Service. See Metcalfe, A.J. (Commonwealth Director-General of Health) to the Minister of Health, March 10, 1949 (A1928, 715/38/1 Section 1), NAA.
60. Whitty, 'The Lepers' Faith,' 211.

61. Henschke to Kerrins, April 29, 1943 (Prov. Corr., N.T. Darwin 1943), MSCK.
62. Kerrins to Henschke, October 14, 1943 (Prov. Corr., N.T. Darwin 1943), MSCK.
63. McCarthy to Kerrins, April 4, 1944 (Prov. Corr., N.T. Darwin 1944), MSCK.
64. Father "Murphy" to Breene, November 9, 1948 (Prov. Corr., N.T. Darwin 1948), MSCK.
65. 'Report of Committee of Inquiry,' part 2, 8, November 19, 1946 (A1928, 715/38/1 Section 3), NAA.
66. Father "Murphy" to Breene, November 9, 1948 (Prov. Corr., N.T. Darwin 1948), MSCK.
67. *Constitution of the Society of Missionaries of the Sacred Heart of Jesus*, Sacred Heart Monastery, Kensington, 1942, no. 4 (f); *Statutes for the Australian Province of the MSC of Jesus*, 1946, LVII, 254a.
68. Various correspondence (Prov. Corr., N.T. Darwin 1948), MSCK.
69. Henschke to Kerrins, n.d and October 2, 1946 (Prov. Corr., N.T. Darwin 1946), MSCK; Father "Murphy" to Kerrins, October 28, 1948 (Prov. Corr., N.T. Darwin 1948), MSCK.
70. Gsell to Kerrins, April 3, 1947 (Prov. Corr., N.T. Darwin 1947), MSCK (N. B. The word 'society' here refers to the MSC religious society).
71. 'Lepers Suffer in Water Cut.' *The Courier-Mail*, October 6, 1949, 5; 'Leprosarium Chief Resigns.' *Sydney Morning Herald*, October 9, 1949, 7.
72. Metcalfe to Inspector, Public Service Board, c. 1955 (A1928, 715/38/1 Section 1), NAA.
73. Metcalfe to O'Loughlin, March 14, 1956 (Prov. Corr., N.T. Darwin 1956), MSCK.
74. Fantome Island priest (name withheld) to Kerrins, August 25, 1941 (Palm Island 1940–1941), MSCK.
75. 'Catholic Missions and the Lepers.' *Catholic Missions*, August 1, 1935, 4.

CHAPTER 9

Leprosy Therapy and Patient Welfare in the Assimilation Era

This chapter examines the positive impact of post-war developments on Australian Indigenous leprosy patients. The focus is mainly, but not exclusively, on the Northern Territory where, in 1955, Channel Island leprosarium was replaced with a mainland institution at East Arm, close to Darwin, bringing improved equipment and accommodation, and decreasing patient isolation. From the late 1940s, the Sisters delivered increasingly efficacious health care due to medical advances and greater participation by specialist doctors. They assumed a wider range of roles, including public education and patient rehabilitation. Drugs developed in the 1940s and continually refined in the ensuing decades, not only radically improved patients' health, but reduced the infectivity of the disease, and discharge from the leprosarium became possible for more Indigenous patients. The extent of reforms across the different leprosaria reflected funding and interest by respective governments. At East Arm, under Commonwealth jurisdiction, they were most pronounced due to the international human rights movement and the avid implementation of the government assimilation policy. But marriages and adoptions of babies arranged earlier by leprosarium staff led to conflicts when patients were discharged. Government authorities applied assimilationist principles to solve them, undercutting traditional law and depriving some people from reuniting with their families.

C. Robson, *Missionary Women, Leprosy and Indigenous Australians, 1936–1986*, https://doi.org/10.1007/978-3-031-05796-0_9

Social, Medical, and Religious Changes in the Post-War Era

After successful research with the sulphone class of drugs at Carville leprosarium in the United States in the 1940s, effective treatment was at long last available to leprosy patients. Promin and Dapsone were the earliest examples of these drugs and they worked by inhibiting the replication of the leprosy bacillus in the body—arresting the disease, rather than curing it. Sulphone treatment could not reverse, but it could prevent, impairments due to nerve damage, such as blindness or claw hand, and it could clear up skin lesions. Importantly for patient welfare, sulphone treatment also reduced or eliminated infectivity, if the drug regimen was followed carefully.[1] These drugs, and other advances that followed in chemotherapy and corrective surgery opened the way for the large-scale discharge of patients, and, potentially, the dismantling of the leprosarium system. In Australia the latter took another three to four decades, as did the care of leprosy patients by Catholic missionary women.

In 1962, in a reference to Christian missionaries and their past treatment of leprosy sufferers, leading international leprologist, Doctor Stanley Browne, commented, "the emotional sentimentalism of a former generation is being replaced by practical help in curing the disease, in preventing the deformities it leads to, and in mitigating its psychological and social consequences."[2] Chapter 5 has argued, rather to the contrary, that in their care of Australian leprosy patients from the 1930s, trained missionary nursing Sisters pursued these same therapeutic objectives in pragmatic and innovative ways, limited only by the meagre resources available to them. But Browne, himself a medical missionary with thirty years' experience with leprosy sufferers in Africa, should not be seen as critical of his fellow workers, as much as optimistic for new possibilities facilitated by the scientific progress of the post-war era. Only in retrospect can we see that it would take more than medical milestones and sincere hard work to wipe away a tarnish of more than two thousand years' duration.

Browne was not the only churchman to reappraise the Christian leprosy apostolate following the advent of the sulphone drugs. In 1951, Pope Pius XII called to account the many Catholic religious involved in this work, stressing the need for professional training and knowledge before embarking on "the fairest flowers of mission endeavour," as he called Catholic leprosy care.[3] At the same time, he acknowledged "the nuns with full professional qualifications who have earned well merited recognition by the special study of loathsome diseases, such as leprosy, and by discovering remedies for them."[4] If his choice of words to describe the disease did nothing to support the force of this appeal, then at least other sections of the Catholic Church in this period, especially those working with patients, were urging the religious to take up the campaign for the de-stigmatisation of leprosy launched by Carville patient, Stanley Stein. Sister Sullivan of Carville advised seminarians not to use the word 'leprosy' as a "synonym for sin" in their sermons.[5]

In the same period, the policy of assimilation for Indigenous people was promoted by all levels of government, bringing with it the promise of equality with white Australians. The Commonwealth government, through its administration of the Northern Territory, was especially proactive in furthering this policy, as articulated in its 1953 Welfare Ordinance, "to promote their social, economic and political advancement for the purpose of assisting them and their descendants to take their place as members of the Commonwealth."[6] Minister for the Territories Paul Hasluck saw the policy as a way "to give the chance of a happy and useful life to all our people."[7] Rhetorically, the policy had a great deal to offer Indigenous leprosy sufferers, as they began to be discharged and rejoin society. In addition, as a founding member of the United Nations (UN), Australia had emerged from the war committed in principle to the support of international human rights. Furthermore, under the umbrella of the UN, the World Health Organisation (WHO) set up the Expert Committee on Leprosy in 1952, publishing the same year its first set of international guidelines for humane and efficacious medical treatment regimes.

The welfare of Australian Indigenous leprosy patients at Derby and Fantome Island, tucked away at the far western and eastern extremities of the continent, escaped much public scrutiny. Not so for East Arm, easily accessible from the town of Darwin, and not far from the airport which, since the war, had become a busy transit point for journalists and politicians. East Arm attracted attention because it was under Commonwealth government control. What went on there could be seen as reflective of the nation's treatment of its most disadvantaged Indigenous inhabitants as indicated in a communication in 1962 from the Commonwealth Department of Territories to the Director-General of Health. Information was required such that "from the international viewpoint it will be shown that aboriginal lepers are treated in a humanitarian way." The Acting Minister for Territories

would like to be able to mention—

a. The education and training given to them so that they can fulfil a useful place in the community;
b. The medical treatment given to them and the prospects of a cure;
c. That adequate facilities exist to give proper medical treatment and training to those handicapped by the complaint.[8]

The pressure to uphold Australia's international reputation for human rights and to further the Commonwealth government's assimilation policy resulted in more funding and resources for East Arm than for the other leprosaria from the 1950s to the 1970s. Consequently, therapeutic reforms and programmes to prepare patients for life outside the institution occurred earlier and more extensively. But at all institutions, the Catholic Sister nurses and the new cohort of medical officers remained committed to their work within the limits imposed by the available resources.

Changes in Nursing and Medical Care

In the early to mid-1950s, many patients, having been stabilised on one or other of the new sulphone class of drugs, began to markedly improve and were increasingly being discharged from the leprosaria. The impact of this therapy was most dramatic at Fantome Island where, before 1948, only two patients had ever been discharged. The population peaked at seventy-seven in early 1949, decreased to sixty-five by 1954 and then, over the following two years, plunged to twenty-six. Furthermore, only a few patients were being admitted each year and the Queensland Director-General of Health, Abraham Fryberg, justifiably predicted that "in a few years' time leprosy will be almost completely eliminated from the coloured population of Queensland."[9] At Derby, reports by the religious Sisters were similarly buoyant as substantial numbers, sometimes over fifty each year, were discharged in the early to mid-1950s. Discharges in the Northern Territory, although remaining modest until the late 1950s, were well above the previous figure of only four in pre-sulphone days. These outcomes engendered optimism among remaining patients: they were the first concrete evidence that the leprosarium was not a life sentence.

Queensland medical officer, Morgan Gabriel, noted on visiting Fantome Island, "...the whole outlook of the coloured patients has altered as the result of modern treatment."[10]

However, not all patients responded well to the new drugs. After their introduction to Indigenous patients in 1947, some had serious, sometimes fatal reactions. Sister Paule, who arrived at Fantome Island in 1948, remembered about six people dying after treatment with Sulphetrone and that "some went wild."[11] At Channel Island, a 12-year-old girl died after developing a severe blood disorder.[12] Dr Gabriel concluded that "the coloured patients do not tolerate any of the drugs in the high dosages needed in white patients."[13] This racial explanation was later countered by a theory that pre-existing anaemias, perhaps due to hookworm, had predisposed Indigenous people to toxic effects. The Queensland health department conceded "the impossibility at present of controlling these reactions."[14] After doctors reduced recommended dosages or introduced newer, less toxic sulphones, most Indigenous patients begin to experience improvements.

The careful administration of the drugs, the constant testing and the management of side-effects left the Sisters little time for tasks other than their clinical duties. The Sisters of St John of God Kimberley Superior noted that extra attention had to be devoted to the individual patient. "The new drug has increased the work for the sisters as the patients who are getting this treatment have to be carefully watched by taking and testing their blood count and also urine testing more frequently to avoid the danger of kidney destruction."[15]

These new demands brought doctors into more regular contact with the Sisters and patients than before, and they became more integral to leprosarium health teams, once almost exclusively the domain of the Sister nurses. Sister Benedicta, who was East Arm leprosarium matron until 1965, stated that having doctors committed to leprosy treatment "was an advance to us...because they had the advantage of belonging to the Health Department and they could see a future for these people, once we got the doctors in."[16] Their greater participation allowed for more rigorous management of treatments, the incorporation of innovations such as new drugs and reconstructive surgery and opportunities to train the Sisters in supporting or administering these treatments. It also brought them face-to-face with the patients' circumstances, with the result that some doctors became advocates for their improved welfare. From the mid-1950s to at least the late 1960s, the senior medical officers attending East Arm, Fantome Island and Derby were, respectively, John Hargrave, Morgan Gabriel, and J.J. Elphinstone. In Western Australia and Queensland, leprosarium work would remain part of the overall work of the medical officer, but in 1963, Hargrave's appointment at East Arm became full time when the position of resident medical superintendent was created.

Hargrave had come to the Northern Territory in the mid-1950s as a young medical survey officer who quickly developed interest and expertise in Indigenous health and, more specifically, in the leprosy outbreaks affecting communities at the time. Mother Marion, East Arm matron between 1959 and 1965, explained how Hargrave's arrival enabled the Sisters to adopt modern and effective leprosy nursing:

> From my point of view, it was a very fortunate occurrence because he was a very good teacher, very good at delegating things, and once he taught you how to do things, he would let you get on and do it. I found myself doing all sorts of things that I never dreamt of doing. Yes, that was a great blessing for me, and therefore the people, because he was really committed very seriously to the work and he was very up to date with what was happening in the leprosy field and embracing everything as it came up and translating it into action in the leprosarium.[17]

This very positive appraisal reveals, first, the harmonious and mutually rewarding working relationship shared by Mother Marion and Hargrave. As intended, it also conveys Hargrave's capabilities for imparting skills and giving the Sisters the confidence to use them, and the medical innovations he brought to East Arm—all of which was to benefit the patients. But, without a closer consideration of Mother Marion's comments, we might miss the essential role she and the Sisters played in carrying out these health interventions. She was, after all, the one who would "get on and do it." The patients' health—sometimes whether they lived or died—depended on the practical application of Hargrave's lessons by the Sister nurses, a task that entailed the day-to-day treatment of hundreds of patients at the bedside, the operating theatre or the clinic. This is not to say Hargrave did not also personally treat and operate on patients, which will be discussed further (Fig. 9.1).

Mother Marion came from generations of Sisters trained to eschew displays of self-importance, so the downplaying of her leprosarium work in her memories is not surprising. However, her time as leprosarium

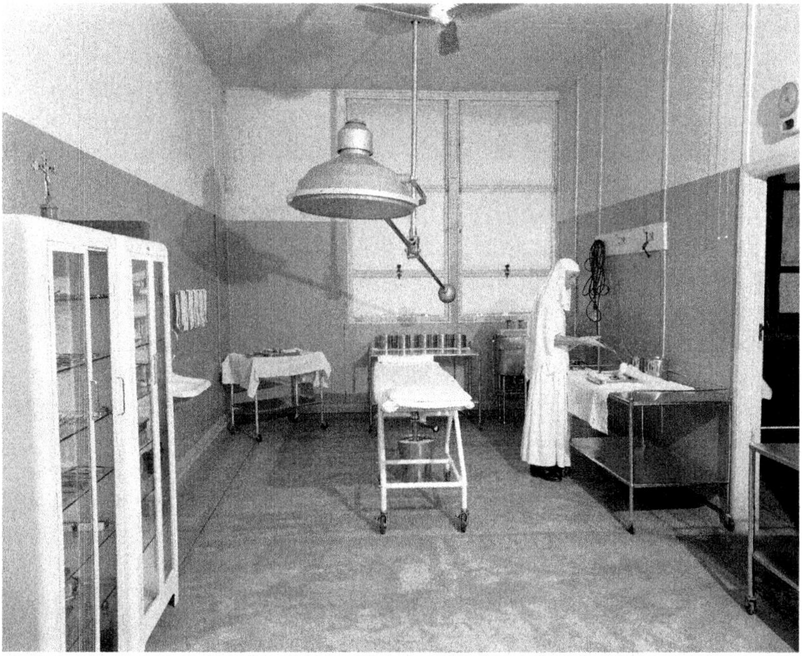

Fig. 9.1 Sister in Surgery, 1958, East Arm Leprosarium (National Archives of Australia)

matron occurred on the cusp of change for women religious, ushered in by the Second Vatican Council. The pressure on Sisters to shroud their identities and achievements in anonymity was lifting, permitting them to expand the professional aspects of their work. The expertise of some leprosarium Sisters in diagnosis and treatment began to be recognised and fostered by health bureaucracies and doctors. East Arm Sisters participated in biomedical research projects at the leprosarium and co-authored medical journal articles.[18] Sister Marion and Derby's Sister Camille gave talks to educate doctors and community members on leprosy, and the latter was sent overseas on a government grant for three months' study at the Carville leprosarium in the USA in 1969.[19] In contrast, fifteen years previously, when Channel Island's Sister Michaeline requested a trip to Fantome Island to observe clinical practices, it was begrudgingly granted as part of her respite trip to Sydney.[20] The Sisters' nursing work was recognised more widely when matrons of all three leprosaria were awarded imperial honours in recognition of their leprosarium nursing.[21]

Years of experience observing the multifarious manifestations of leprosy—a disease that is "unique with respect to the infinite variety of the host response to bacterial invasion"—and training by doctors had made the Sisters some of the few skilled diagnosticians in Australia.[22] Sr Camille was an expert in diagnosing cases of tuberculoid leprosy, a type that can severely damage peripheral nerves.[23] It is easily confused with a range of other (non-leprous) conditions and its presence cannot be confirmed by bacteriological tests.[24] Thus misdiagnoses of the disease made by unqualified people in an earlier period resulted in unnecessary long-term stays at leprosaria. In the early-1970s Sister Camille was regularly flown on leprosy surveys in the Kimberley in this capacity and positive cases were returned with her to the leprosarium.

But her poignant reminiscences indicate that, in the context of the policy of compulsory isolation for leprosy sufferers, her ability was indeed an unenviable distinction, since a positive clinical diagnosis could lead to the immediate separation of a person from his or her family.

> To pick up the cases early was very important. We would bring them in straight away if positive. Once we had to separate a mother from her baby when we diagnosed her leprosy. It was awful, but although we were supposed to take her straight away, I waited for a while so she had some time with her before she had to go.[25]

For decades, the Sisters had been distant from this aspect of policy, an experience that at the hands of police had been often demeaning and frightening for both the patients and the families they left behind.

Rehabilitation

Among the innovations introduced by Hargrave to East Arm, was the supply of prostheses to patients with loss or partial loss of limbs from 1958. The Commonwealth government had been supplying artificial limbs to returned servicemen in Australia since World War I yet there had been no arrangement in place for leprosy sufferers until this time.[26] Fittingly, it was from one of the Department of Repatriation's artificial limb factories that Hargrave, with the support of Northern Territory Health Director, Richard Webb, obtained the prostheses. After

Hargrave underwent training in measuring, ordering, and fitting, he taught the Sisters to do the same, and, a few years later, a workshop for the manufacture of prostheses and surgical boots was set up at the leprosarium.[27]

In 1958, Hargrave, again with Webb's backing, began the expansion of physiotherapy services for the prevention and treatment of deformities caused by nerve damage. The Commonwealth government approved visits of a physiotherapist for one afternoon a week during which she just had time to provide some treatment and to give instruction to the Sisters so that they could continue the work the rest of the time. But this was insufficient to treat 180 patients, two-thirds of whom Webb estimated required more intensive therapy "owing to the severe and often neglected nature of the lesions."[28] Certain of these lesions, if not treated, resulted in "wasting, paresis, paralysis, abnormal gait or stance, eventually contractures and irreversible deformity."[29] Webb invoked the Commonwealth government's assimilation policy when he applied for a full-time physiotherapist for East Arm:

> A settlement such as East Arm Settlement where a patient may well spend years, affords an opportunity probably unrivalled in the Northern Territory to educate and train the more intelligent native in trades and crafts – provided the physical lesions are dealt with first – it is therefore up to the Department of Health to show a lead and do everything in its power to provide a physical basis for vocational rehabilitation and indeed training.[30]

The Commonwealth Director-General, however, thought the suggestion "a little premature"; it would suffice to make a "start on physiotherapy" with groups sessions supervised by the Sisters[31] (Fig. 9.2).

In 1962, Hargrave took up a fellowship granted by WHO to study corrective surgery techniques under Paul Brand at the Christian Medical College in India.[32] As a result, from 1963, operations to repair crippling deformities of the hands and feet became available. By the middle of 1966, most patients had undergone surgical procedures, 179 separate operations having been conducted in the preceding financial year. In 1964, corrective surgery was also begun at Derby leprosarium by Lawson Holman. With the surgery, as with the prosthetics and physiotherapy, the Sisters acquired more specialisation, becoming theatre nurses and research assistants.

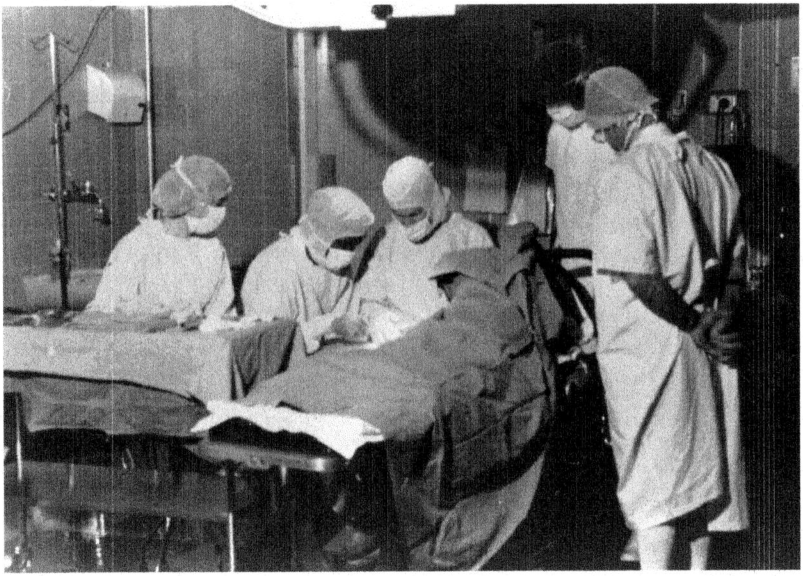

Fig. 9.2 'Operating theatre, East Arm 1977' (Charles Darwin University Nursing Museum)

Physiotherapy, both post- and pre-operatively, was a vital adjunct to this surgery. As neither East Arm nor Derby had qualified physiotherapists at this stage, the leprosarium nursing Sisters took over the role after appropriate training.[33] One Sister at East Arm, who was the first to perform this work, remembered the effect on one patient after surgery to repair claw hand, a deformity which paralyses the hands and makes grasping objects difficult or impossible:

> ...when they had the surgery, they had to do exercises to keep their joints moving. One man who was sitting up in the front seat during midnight Mass with his arms raised high was doing his exercises all during the Holy Mass. You could see this man—he was just so proud of his hands—he wanted everybody to see them.[34]

Holman also noted the patients' response to surgery at Derby where "the possession of a surgically reconstructed hand has become a status symbol."[35]

Corrective surgery was valuable to the patients themselves and it was also seen as of value to the leprosy control programme. It restored function, enabling resumption of work and other activities, and it boosted the patients' self-confidence because of the improvement to their appearance. It was also one of the only measures that could send a positive message to Indigenous communities about the treatment at the leprosarium, and thus potentially induce those evading treatment to come forward. European medicine seemed rather a failure when patients were discharged with permanent disfigurement, even if their infection had been brought under control. As one patient from Fantome Island told an interviewer regarding sulphone therapy: "Oooh, it wasn't a real cure, you know. They go there real good, like you, and they come out something wrong with them. No I don't think it was a real cure."[36]

An important role assumed by the leprosarium Sisters was the training of Indigenous health assistants. From the outset, the Sisters at all institutions had taught the patients, usually the women, to do simple tasks such as make and autoclave the dressings, to lighten their own workloads and provide therapeutic occupations.[37] From the mid-1950s, East Arm Sisters began to train some patients in laboratory and assistant nursing duties, facilitated by the new equipment installed after the move from Channel Island. Patients were taught to analyse tissue samples under the microscope, give injections and excise small ulcers.[38] Trained patients then carried out these tasks as employees of the leprosarium. As with so many developments in the leprosarium in this period, the scheme was considered in terms of its value to the discharged patient and was acclaimed by the Director of Health as a significant contribution towards the government's objective "of training natives to become useful members of society."[39]

This scheme was the forerunner of the 'paramedicals' programme initiated by Hargrave in the 1960s. Paramedicals were trained Indigenous personnel working among their own communities, diagnosing leprosy and providing basic treatment. In 1960, WHO recommended the employment of paramedicals for local leprosy campaigns as they enabled outpatient treatment, thereby minimising the trauma and disruption to life caused by leprosarium isolation. [40] In a conversation with the author in 2011, Hargrave explained that he thought it important to transfer some areas of treatment from the control of European to Indigenous workers, to not only further the paramedicals' own prospects as skilled workers, but also to temper what had for so long been a hard-handed approach to leprosy control. After he enlisted the support of the Director of Welfare and various mission bodies, the government provided training grants in 1969 and an eight-month course was set up for students, mainly consisting of former leprosy patients.[41]

In the 1960s, some East Arm staff became educators of the public in a campaign to reduce the stigma attached to leprosy. Patients discharged from the leprosarium often experienced prejudice as they went about trying to remake their lives out of isolation. They had to continue their medication and therefore were not infectious but nevertheless, as Sharon McGregor's study has revealed, they were barred from training courses and employment, particularly in the town of Darwin.[42] Northern Territory psychiatrist, John Cawte, who treated former patients, observed a pattern of detrimental psychological and physical consequences of this stigma.[43] In 1962, the incarceration of two patients at Fanny Bay Jail sparked a public controversy when wardens refused to guard them, and locals aired their complaints in the newspaper. 'Puzzled of Parap' wrote,

> It is all very well for Dr Byrne to say there is little health risk in looking after leprosy sufferers and to point out that the wonderful nuns of East Arm and doctors who treat them don't catch the disease. These people know exactly what they are doing and what to look for. Anyway it is their choice. If leprosy isn't contagious why lock them up anyway?[44]

Against this background, staff tried to defuse panic and confusion by disseminating information in government publications, newspapers and public speeches.[45] Mother Marion gave presentations to the Darwin Country Women's Association (CWA), the Rotary Club, and MSC seminarians. She remembers feeling overwhelmed at the unexpectedly large audience at the CWA function. When asked the subject of this speech, she replied, "I told them about leprosy and I told them about things they needn't be worried about and the things that maybe they should be worried about. That's all"[46] (Fig. 9.3).

Another facet of the staff's public relations exercise was the de-stigmatisation of the leprosarium itself. Its reputation as a place of long-term strict confinement invoked terror in Indigenous communities, sending those who suspected they were infected into the bush rather than come forward for help. Despite advances in leprosy therapy, however, Indigenous people in the late-1960s were still fearful of the leprosarium.[47] Staff wanted them to know about effective medicine and

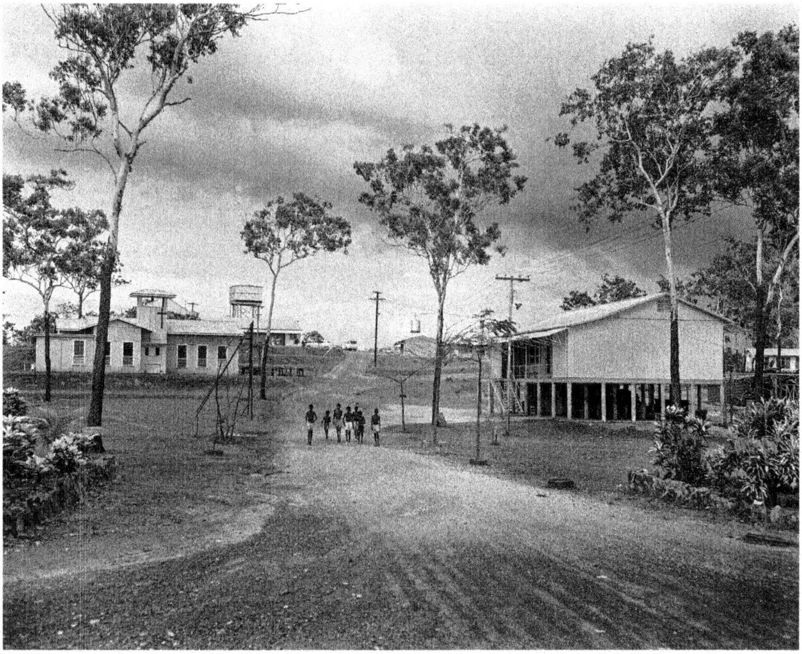

Fig. 9.3 East Arm Leprosarium, Darwin, 1958 (National Archives of Australia)

that patients were no longer kept for decades in isolation. To avoid treatment was, in this new era, to invite a tragic outcome. Furthermore, as the anti-segregation brigade had warned many years previously, avoidance only heightened the risk of infecting others. Inspired by similar action overseas, administrators at East Arm decided to dispense with the term 'leprosarium' in the name of the institution and to instead call it the 'East Arm Settlement,' thus eliminating negative connotations that might discourage voluntary admissions.[48]

Financial Remuneration of the Sisters

How, if at all, were these shifting roles measured in the financial remuneration paid by governments for the Sisters' services? By 1949, the subsidy paid to their communities for their work was about £4 per week per Sister across all three institutions. These amounts bore no relation to the Sisters' individual qualifications, the hours worked or duties performed. In 1951, the provincial superiors of both the Daughters of Our Lady of the Sacred Heart and the Franciscan Missionaries of Mary (FMM) applied to have this situation remedied. The Queensland government increased the Fantome Sisters' subsidy and apportioned it according to their qualifications. The matron, two nursing Sisters and two others (whose duties included teaching, looking after supplies, and other general tasks), received £12, £10 and £6 per week, respectively. They also received £400 per annum for food, two return airfares to Brisbane for the matron, as well as free board and lodging.[49]

The DOLSH Sisters' application was less successful. The superior had asked for the rate paid to regular nurses of the Northern Territory Medical Service: an "infectious nursing allowance" plus remuneration corresponding to the midwifery qualifications and the seniority of the sister-in-charge. However, the Catholic Bishop of Darwin, John O'Loughlin, weighed in on the discussion, declaring this method of remuneration was "not in keeping with the religious vocation of the missionaries, nor does it reflect adequately the true relationship of the Mission to the Department of Health."[50] The government took his advice and approved a modest rise to £6.10 for each Sister.

The superiors' push for their Sisters to be recognised on the same financial basis as regular nursing Sisters—however inadequate—indicates that they now considered they had more leverage with the government. Successful treatments in the 1950s could be tied directly to their nursing. Its greater focus on the individual patient and his/her transition to recovery and discharge, rather than the more custodial and generalised care of previous years, resembled general hospital nursing. However, for the Derby Sisters, the per capita system continued at least until 1970, with small incremental rises in the rate over the years.

The superiors' 1951 applications for differential rates were given added impetus by gains made in the Australian nursing industry generally in the latter part of the 1940s, such as the 44-hour week and higher awards. After improvements in nurses' conditions and wages in the 1920s, they had remained either stable or regressed over the austere years of the Depression and the Second World War due, according to Glenda Strachan, to attitudes among nurses' associations and doctors that "nursing was built on self-sacrifice" and that therefore, it was "hard to request wages or shorter working hours."[51] Post-war reform only occurred because of an acute nurse shortage, highlighted by nurses' industrial action.[52] Against this broader context, the reasons for Bishop O'Loughlin's veto can be clarified. In his eyes, quantifying the religious Sisters' nursing work in monetary terms diminished its self-sacrificial dimension and derogated the Sisters to the status of government secular nurses. The difference, implied by O'Loughlin in a public speech in 1957, was in the Catholic Sisters' religious motivation: while secular medicine "may attempt to alleviate the suffering of these lepers," the religious Sisters provided spiritual healing in which "pain [could be] accepted in the Christian spirit."[53] His near-denial of the Sisters' professionalism was therefore at odds with the view of the provincial superiors, who, having charge over nurses in missions and Catholic hospitals, knew full well that efficacious nursing services at low cost were being supplied to government leprosaria over which the Church had little control.

In 1966, the DOLSH again applied for their subsidy to be aligned with regular nurses' wages. Mother Anthony, the East Arm superior argued that their nursing had become more specialised, and that the last increase, to £8.10 ($17 in decimal currency), had been in 1955.[54] Eight Sisters nursed 101 patients whereas at Fantome Island, three Sisters received $30 and the Matron, $34, for looking after just six patients, while at Derby the rate was $22 per Sister.[55] Again, Bishop O'Loughlin's opinion was sought and sustained. He recommended continuing on the same basis as "the value of the services rendered by the Sisters depends on their efficiency as a group more than on their individual qualifications" and that a $5 increase was sufficient, to take effect in December 1966.[56] It was not until 1974 that the East Arm Sisters' nursing qualifications were reflected in the remuneration while at the same time the amounts finally matched those of regular nurses.

New Controls Under the Guise of Assimilation

As part of the new assimilation policy of the mid-1950s, the Northern Territory government began to assume more direct responsibility for leprosy patients, through its Welfare Branch, the department created for overseeing policy. Welfare officers, patrolling their allotted districts implemented the Welfare Ordinance of 1953 under the authority of their divisional head, were charged with looking after the rights of the patients and ensuring they had some choices about their lives and those of their children, thus challenging the hegemonic control of the Catholic missionaries. The officers were the successors to the less formal patrol officers introduced soon after World War II, who had regularly visited Channel Island from the late-1940s, to deal with individual concerns of the patients. They had reconnected some patients with their former communities by organising visits from friends and relatives, and conveying letters and photographs between the parties.[57] Initially, the religious Brother who was the leprosarium superintendent was unwelcoming and regarded their visits as a departmental check on the Catholic missionaries' management.[58] In a way he was correct as, with the more intensive monitoring by officers of the Welfare Branch, who were newly educated in Professor Elkin's course in anthropology at Sydney University, many of the restrictions that characterised patient management under religious and lay authorities began to be unravelled.

By 1959, some of the policies at the East Arm were reviewed, due to issues facing patients on their discharge from the leprosarium. The meeting to decide on the new set of procedures consisted of welfare officers, the medical officer, and the Director of Health. Catholic missionaries, once always a part of such decision-making, were notably not included. One principle that was agreed upon was that actions concerning the patients should not be coercive but should be based on the cooperation of the patient, including when dealing with people who evaded treatment. The welfare officer was to try to convince the person that treatment was in their best interests and to "induce the patient to accompany him" to the leprosarium. Police were only to be used as a last resort.[59] Similarly, rules drawn up for leprosarium staff at the same time outlawed corporal punishment and provided for the establishment of a committee of elders, drawn from the patient population, for discussing problems and suggesting punishments for offences. The committee had little decision-making power, however, as it met under the "guidance" of the medical and lay superintendents.[60]

Under the new provisions, welfare officers were charged with finding appropriate foster care for babies born to patients with consideration to be given to "the return of the child to the parents after they are discharged, and the location of the parents on resettlement."[61] This rule formalised what had been occurring in the previous few years. For example, in 1955, Patrol Officer Egan, after interviews with two expectant mothers, overturned the plan to send their babies to the Catholic Mission on Bathurst Island and arranged, instead, for their transfer to their mothers' home countries, Oenpelli and Roper River, to be cared for by aunts.[62]

To understand the ramifications of the older arrangements, it is helpful to look briefly at the case of a couple from the Anglican mission at Oenpelli whose four children, born at Channel Island between 1947 and 1952, were fostered out to Catholic mission families on Bathurst Island, as had been customary. After their discharge from the leprosarium, the parents tried unsuccessfully to regain custody of the three younger girls and return them to Oenpelli. In 1965, with legal channels recently opened to them under provisions of the new Social Welfare Ordinance (NT), they took their case to the Supreme Court but this action and the subsequent appeal failed, mainly on the grounds of disruption to the girls'

> deeply rooted bonds of family devotion and friendships and other personal interests and ambitions, all of which are confined to Bathurst Island, their disinterest in their natural parents, and the probabilities of serious injury to health and lasting unhappiness being caused to any of them being moved to Oenpelli...[63]

The case elucidates the extent of the rift that was wrought between family members through fostering out children to locations with different cultures to those of their parents. The children, raised on Bathurst Island, had learnt Tiwi language and were unable to converse with their natural parents; they had adopted the Catholic faith, whereas their parents were Protestant; and they had been integrated into Tiwi skin groupings and promised to compatible men as brides.[64]

In determining that the parents had consented in the first place to their children's removal to Bathurst Island, the judge justified and sustained the same practice that the welfare officers had been trying to eliminate over the previous decade. He based his view that consent had been given, first, on the absence of any evidence that the parents opposed or tried to prevent the removal, and second because the father had "handed each of three girls to an adult for escort to the Bathurst Island mission."[65] As is clear from Chapter 7, this version of the standard child removal procedure is patently false. The parents were not permitted to touch their infant; for removal to take place, the Sister had to lift the newborn and then carry him/her away from the mother. It is doubtful that as Indigenous leprosarium patients, the parents would have been able to provide or withhold informed consent, as was appreciated by the Director of Welfare who in 1960 cautioned an officer, "I cannot emphasise too much that the interviewing officer must be satisfied that whatever consent [the patient] gives in respect of the future of her child must be given completely willingly and without any pressure to bear."[66]

One positive result to emerge from this legal fight was a change in policy in 1966 regarding the future fostering of Australian leprosarium babies.[67] New guidelines were issued stipulating that the parents were to decide where the child was to be placed, that they must retain legal guardianship of the child, and that the foster parents must return the child to the natural parents if they asked for custody. A written request by the parents to the nominated custodian was to be made. The parents were to be fully informed of their legal rights by a departmental officer before the placement of the child occurred.[68]

Another procedure endorsed in the 1959 meeting was for the welfare officers, before giving permission for marriage between those classified as wards, to investigate their backgrounds to avoid conflict when they were later discharged. Again, this practice had already been in place since 1956 after a stabbing occurred over the breach of a marriage promise.[69] In the days when discharge from the leprosarium seemed improbable, neither tribal law forbidding unions between people of certain groups nor pre-existing marriage promises had held force in marriages arranged by the Catholic missionaries. As discharges increased, however, some patients were returning to the outside world facing unhappy consequences of these contraventions.

Yet it was not the intention of the Welfare Branch to uphold traditional Indigenous laws, especially if at risk of jeopardising marriages between educated and Christianised men and women; this would run against the grain of its espoused assimilation principles. Instead, in dealing with potentially problematic marriages between parties of different backgrounds, officers were told to look for solutions, and to negotiate with, and prepare "relatives and other 'interested' parties."[70] It seemed, then, that the only change from previous practices was to introduce a diplomatic, supposedly culturally respectful protocol to procure these other parties' agreement to the Christian marriages.

In 1961, welfare officers investigated an application for marriage from a young couple at Port Keats Catholic Mission. The woman had been discharged from East Arm Leprosarium five years previously, but she had not been sent home to Auvergne Station, presumably under health department policy at the time to discharge patients only to areas supplied with nursing services. On investigation, the welfare officers found that her parents opposed the marriage as the woman had been promised to a local man since childhood. Officer E.C. Evans recommended overruling the parents, reasoning,

> by virtue of her training at the Leprosarium and followed up by her education... at Port Keats [she] would be well ahead by Western standards of her relatives back at Auvergne....I do not know who this proposed husband is but he may even be a native who already has a wife or wives. We are faced with an attitude by a female ward which is contrary to the wishes of her parents but which is in fact the development of an ideal in respect of the choosing of partners and the concept of married life which we wish to encourage.[71]

The welfare officers attempted to bring all the parties together at Auvergne, anticipating that the parents might consider the marriage if they could meet the couple. The promised husband, it was thought, could be placated by reimbursement of the bride money he had been paying the parents. Negotiations proceeded no further, however, as it was discovered that the promised husband had recently married the woman's sister.[72]

Bishop O'Loughlin was concerned that female patients who had been baptised Catholic in the leprosarium would be forced to enter arranged marriages if they were discharged somewhere other than the Catholic missions.[73] Beginning with his predecessor, F.X. Gsell, who circumvented Tiwi marriage law on Bathurst Island by "buying" promised brides from their parents, the Catholic missionaries had continued, wherever they had influence, to try to suppress what they saw as barbaric Indigenous practices and to encourage Christian marriage.[74] O'Loughlin, however, was reassured by the Welfare Branch that "provided they did not have an affiliation with other Missions, the girls may exercise their free will in the matter of religious faith and that if they require the support of this Branch in declining to marry their promised or tribal husbands, then the support would be forthcoming."[75] State and Church, then, worked together to continue the processes of Western Christian assimilation begun in the leprosarium. Long-term institutionalisation in such cases alienated the leprosy patients from their culture and their family, irrevocably.

* * *

This chapter has demonstrated that by the middle of the 1950s, conditions were optimised in Australia for setting Indigenous leprosy sufferers on the road to recovery from their disease, correction of their disabilities, and reinstatement to their home communities with, if necessary, government financial support. It has shown that, as far as possible, the Catholic nursing Sisters along with the doctors worked to achieve these ends. In this period, senior Sisters became recognised experts in leprosy care, trained Indigenous health assistants and survey nurses, were involved in conducting clinical research, and provided public education to try to reduce leprosy stigma. The vigorous attention by the Commonwealth government in the Northern Territory to the assimilation policy saw a shift in authority by the Catholic Church over patient lives to government agencies. In many ways, however, the paternalistic control of the Catholic missionaries was simply transferred to the Welfare Branch and continued to reflect disdain for Indigenous traditions and the people's capacity for self-determination.

Notes

1. Robson, Charmaine. 2016. 'Ending Isolation? Leprosy, Welfare and Indigenous Australians 1950–86.' *Aboriginal History* 40, 69.
2. Browne, S.G. 1962. 'Leprosy: The Christian Attitude,' *The Expository Times* 73, 242.
3. Pope Pius XII. 'Evangelii Praecones,' Vatican, 1951 (Accessed March 15, 2010) http://www.vatican.va/holy_father/pius_xii/encyclicals/documents/hf_p-xii_enc_02061951_evangelii-praecones_en.html, s. 45.
4. Ibid., s. 47.
5. Sullivan, Sr Catherine quoted in Brown, Raphael. 1951. *World Survey of Catholic Leprosy Work*. Techny, Illinois: The Mission Press, 33.
6. Parliament of the Commonwealth of Australia, 1956. *Report on the Administration of the Northern Territory, 1953–1955*. Canberra: Government of the Commonwealth of Australia, 37.
7. Cited in McGregor, Russell. 2011. *Indifferent Inclusion, Aboriginal People and the Australian Nation*. Canberra: Aboriginal Studies Press, 78.
8. Secretary, Department of Territories to Director-General, November 9, 1962 (A1658, 756/11/1 PART 2), National Archives of Australia (NAA).
9. Queensland Health and Medical Services Branch. 1957. *Annual Report on the Health and Medical Services of the State of Queensland 1955–1956*. Brisbane: The State, 19.
10. Queensland Health and Medical Services Branch. 1958. *Annual Report on the Health and Medical Services of the State of Queensland 1956–1957*. Brisbane: The State, 17.

11. Duford, Sister Paule. 198_. Interview with Siobhan McHugh. Siobhan McHugh Collection of Australian Social History. Sound recording (ORALTRC 2761/5). National Library of Australia (NLA).
12. Kettle, Ellen. 1991. *Health Services in the Northern Territory: A History 1824–1970,* volume two. Darwin: North Australia Research Unit, 44.
13. Gabriel, Morgan. 1955. 'Report on a Visit to Fantome Island- July 1955,' 1, (Director of Native Affairs Office, GF/1, Correspondence, Aboriginal and Torres Strait Islander, ID ITM714733), Queensland State Archives (QSA).
14. Queensland Health and Medical Services Branch. 1952. *Annual Report on the Health and Medical Services of the State of Queensland 1950–1951*, Brisbane: The State, 8.
15. Extracts from Visitation of Provincials and Generals 1937–1976, April 6, 1951 (2.621), Sisters of St John of God Archives Broome (SSJGB).
16. Carroll, Sister Benedicta OLSH. Interview with author. Typed transcript. Recorded at DOLSH Convent, Kensington, New South Wales, September 9, 2008.
17. Whelan, Sister Marion OLSH. Interview with author. Typed transcript. Recorded at DOLSH Convent, Kensington, New South Wales, August 12, 2008.
18. Marion, Reverend Mother. 1965. 'New Approach to Old Problem.' Australian Territories, Canberra: Department of Territories, 5 (6), 31–38; Hargrave, J.C. and Marion, Reverend Mother. 1964. 'Leprotic Involvement of Multiple Peripheral Nerves in the Absence of Skin Lesions.' *Leprosy Review* 35, 78–82; McLeod, J.G., J.C. Hargrave, J.C. Walsh, G.C. Booth, R. Gye and Sister Annette Barron. 1975. 'Nerve Conduction Studies in Leprosy,' *International Journal of Leprosy* 43, 21–31.
19. Carroll, Sr Benedicta. Interview with author; 'Information on Sisters 1968–1971,' (2.47 K), SSJGB; Walsh, Sister Lorna quoted in Gardiner, Anne. 2008. *The Flame in the North: The Daughters of Our Lady of the Sacred Heart 1908–2008*. Darwin: the author, 49.
20. Mugavin, Michaeline, Sr to Metcalfe, A.J. (Commonwealth Director-General of Health). October 1954 (A1658, 756/11/3 PART 1), NAA.
21. Gertrude Greene, 1948; Alphonsus Daly, 1958; Irma St Nérée, 1965; Marion Whelan, 1962. See Faith, Hope and Charity: Australian Women and Imperial Honours 1901–1989. http://www.womenaustralia.info/exhib/honours/g.html; http://www.womenaustralia.info/exhib/honours/d.html; http://www.womenaustralia.info/exhib/honours/n.html; http://www.womenaustralia.info/exhib/honours/m.html Accessed 3 December 2021.
22. 'Leprosy Over the Last 25 Years,' *Medical Journal of Australia*, October 1, 1972, 801.

23. Poidevin, Sister Camille SJG. Interview with author. Typed transcript. Recorded at Derby, Western Australia, 17 November 2008.
24. Hargrave, J.C. 1968. *Leprosy in Northern Territory Aborigines: A Short Guide for Nursing Sisters in the Diagnosis, Treatment and Management of Leprosy in Aborigines*. Darwin: Northern Territory Medical Service, 15, 17.
25. Poidevin, Sr Camille. Interview with author.
26. Bourke, Joanna. 1998. 'The Battle of the Limbs: Amputation, Artificial Limbs and the Great War in Australia.' *Australian Historical Studies* 29 (110), 54, 56.
27. Kettle, *Health Services*, 50; Parliament of the Commonwealth of Australia, 1961. *Report on the Administration of the Northern Territory, 1959–1960*. Canberra: Government of the Commonwealth of Australia, 38.
28. Webb, Richard (Northern Territory Director to Health) to Metcalfe, February 7, 1958. (A1658, 756/11/3 PART 1), NAA.
29. Ibid.
30. Ibid.
31. Acting Commonwealth Director-General of Health to Webb, January 30, 1958 (A1658, 756/11/3 PART 1), NAA.
32. Hargrave, J.C. 1963. 'International Leprosy Expert Visits Northern Territory' (A1658, 756/11/1 PART 2), NAA.
33. "Sr Helen" OLSH (real name withheld). Interview with author. Typed transcript. Recorded at DOLSH Convent, Kensington, New South Wales, August 18, 2008, Western Australia Public Health Department. 1966. *Report of the Commissioner of Public Health*. Perth: Department of Public Health, 65.
34. "Sr Helen," Interview with author.
35. Western Australia Public Health Department. 1966. *Report of the Commissioner*, 65.
36. Boyd, Sandy. 198–? Interview with Siobhan McHugh, Siobhan McHugh Collection of Australian Social History. Sound recording (ORAL TRC 2761/5). NLA.
37. Sr Benedicta. Interview with author.
38. Brauer. 'A New Look at East Arm'; "Sister Helen." Interview; Sister Marion. Interview.
39. Humphry, A.H. (Northern Territory Director of Health) to Metcalfe. March 1, 1957 (A1658, 756/11/3 PART 1), NAA.
40. World Health Organisation. 1953. 'Expert Committee on Leprosy: Second Report,' *World Health Organisation Technical Report Series,* No.189. Geneva: World Health Organisation, whqlibdoc.who.int/trs/WHO_trs_189.pdf, accessed September 14, 2010, 16–17.

41. Commonwealth Department of the Interior. 1972. *Northern Territory Report 1971–72*. Canberra: Australian Government Printer, 78.
42. McGregor, Sharon. 2004. 'Lepers Can't Change Their Spots.' *Journal of Northern Territory History*, 15, 39–41.
43. Cawte, John. 2001. *Healers of Arnhem Land*. Marleston: J.B. Books, 58–67.
44. 'Puzzled of Parap' to the Editor. *Northern Territory News*. October 27, 1962.
45. E.g. Marion and Hargrave. 'New Approach to Old Problem,' 31–38.
46. Whelan, Sister Marion. Interview with author.
47. Western Australia Public Health Department. 1969. *Report of the Commissioner of Public Health*. Perth: Department of Public Health, 59.
48. Hargrave, John to Langsford, William (Northern Territory Director of Health). June 4, 1964 (E51, 1965/771), NAA.
49. Director of Health (Northern Territory) to Refshauge, William (Commonwealth Director-General of Health). August 4, 1961 (A1658, 756/11/3 PART 3), NAA. At that time, the basic wage for Queensland women was £5.16, and the maximum rate for a senior "Grade 2" nursing sister was £6.2 (also with free board and lodging). See Government Statistician. 1953. *Queensland Year Book No.13, 1952*. Brisbane: Government Statistician's Office, 327, 330.
50. O'Loughlin, Bishop John to Metcalfe. August 10, 1951 (A1658, 756/11/3 PART 3), NAA.
51. Strachan, Glenda. 1991. 'Sacred Office, Trade or Profession: The Dilemma of Nurses' Involvement in Industrial Activities in Queensland.' *Labour History* 61, 162.
52. Ibid., 159–160.
53. O'Loughlin, Bishop John at opening of East Arm Leprosarium Catholic Church quoted in Flynn, Frank. 1963. *Northern Gateway*. Sydney: F.P. Leonard, 24.
54. Anthony, Mother Mary to Langsford. March 8, 1966 (A1658, 756/11/3 PART 3), NAA.
55. Deputy Commonwealth Director-General of Health to Langsford, August 26, 1966, (A1658, 756/11/3 PART 3), NAA.
56. O'Loughlin to Langsford, October 14, 1966 (A1658, 756/11/3 PART 3), NAA.
57. Reports by Patrol Officers: Gordon Sweeney, March 15, June 1, March 16, 1949 and Ted Egan, July 16, 1954 (F1, 1952/526), NAA.
58. Patrol Officer Greenfield to Acting Director, Department of Native Affairs, January 19, 1954 (F1, 1952/526), NAA.
59. 'Marriages of Patients at East Arm Leprosarium' in 'Reports on Discussions between Welfare Branch and Department of Health on Wishes Relating to Leprosy Patients.' August 25, 1959 (F1, 1963/1615), NAA.

60. 'Statement of Responsibilities and Duties at East Arm Leprosarium, August 1959' (E51, 1959/369), NAA.
61. 'Procedural Arrangements for Care of Children born to couples living at East Arm Leprosarium' in Reports on Discussions' (F1, 1963/1615), NAA.
62. Egan to District Welfare Officer, November 1, 1955 (F1, 1955/740), NAA.
63. Bridge, J. 1982. 'Judgment: R.V. Silvester Pilimapitjimiri, Simona Tampulureimulla, Dick Mirringmautimiri and Mary Torramura; ex parte Frank Gananggu and Elsie Darrbuma,' Supreme Court, Darwin, no. 148 of 1965 in *A Selection of the Judgements of the Supreme Court of the Northern Territory of Australia, 1951–1976*, Canberra: Australian Government Printing Service, 786–787.
64. Ibid., 779.
65. Ibid., 777.
66. Director, Department of Welfare to District Welfare Officer, 1960 (F1, 1959/975), NAA.
67. Tatz, Colin. 1979. 'Access to Civil Law.' *Legal Services Bulletin* 4 (5), 198.
68. Commissioner of Native Welfare. 'Derby Leprosarium—Care of Inmates' Children,' August 1, 1966. (DCW 2625, Cons. 1417). State Records Office Western Australia.
69. Director, Department of Welfare to Humphry, April 26, 1956; Humphry to Director, Department of Welfare, May 11, 1956 (F1, 1954/321), NAA.
70. 'Marriages of Patients at East Arm Leprosarium,' Reports on Discussions' (F1, 1963/1615), NAA.
71. Chief Welfare Officer to Director, Department of Welfare, June 12, 1961 (F1, 1959/975), NAA.
72. Patrol Officer Ted Milliken to Chief Welfare Officer, July 31, 1961 (F1, 1959/975), NAA.
73. Humphry to Director, Department of Welfare, May 11, 1956; Chief Welfare Officer E.C. Evans to Sweeney. 1956. (F1, 1954/321), NAA.
74. Gsell, F.X. 1956. *The Bishop with 150 Wives: Fifty Years as a Missionary*. Sydney: Angus and Robertson, 90–91.
75. Evans to Sweeney, 1956. (F1, 1954/321), NAA.

CHAPTER 10

Confinement and Control in the Middle to Late Twentieth Century

The medical advances of the 1950s and 1960s had brought bright prospects for leprosy patients. The positive responses of many Indigenous patients suggested that strict isolation policies would be soon discarded and that they would return to home and families, and resume lives. Similarly, newly diagnosed sufferers might never again be subjected to long-term detention. However, while this scenario played out for most European patients, hardline policies including leprosarium isolation remained in place for Indigenous people until the 1970s and 1980s, due to structural inequities in health care and racialised medical discourse. Whereas medical reforms and high standard facilities were incorporated at East Arm, as Chapter 9 has discussed, governments failed to maintain or upgrade buildings, equipment, and basic services at Derby and Fantome Island, impinging on the health and welfare of the patients. The restrictions and paternalism of continued isolation led to discontent and frustration by an increasingly healthy and socially aware patient population. This chapter examines these consequences of prolonged isolation under these variable conditions and agitation by the religious staff, doctors, and patients for change.

C. Robson, *Missionary Women, Leprosy and Indigenous Australians, 1936–1986*, https://doi.org/10.1007/978-3-031-05796-0_10

A Bifurcated Leprosy Policy

As a result of encouraging results overseas, new guidelines for the management of leprosy sufferers developed by leprologists in the 1950s, were presented at international congresses and prompted the formation of the World Health Organisation's (WHO) Expert Committee on Leprosy in 1952. The first report of the Committee announced that the new treatment "calls for a reconsideration of existing practices regarding compulsory isolation."[1] It recommended first, that only "infectious cases needed to be subjected to some form of isolation, while all cases require treatment" and that infectivity was most reliably established using bacteriological testing, specifically the 'smear' method.[2] Second, the Committee expressed its opposition to compulsory isolation due to its failure in the past to inhibit the spread of the disease by deterring patients from coming forward for treatment. This policy was also considered detrimental to family relationships and to the financial welfare of patients' dependents. The Committee concluded that "the old idea that leprosy is so infectious that patients must be segregated in a distant place is one to be deprecated."[3]

Australian health authorities were unwilling to fully adopt these recommendations. In 1950, the Tropical Hygiene and Medicine Committee of the National Health and Medical Research Council (NHMRC) issued a resolution, restated in 1958, and followed in the case of most Indigenous leprosy sufferers until the 1970s and, for some, the 1980s: "The time is not yet ripe in Australia for abandoning the present prophylactic system. It is in the interest alike of the patient and the general public that all cases of leprosy should be isolated and placed under treatment if necessary in special hospitals."[4] However, also as a result of the 1950 meeting, the Committee began to unravel the more stringent conditions for European leprosy sufferers, as well as for part Indigenous people "regarded as white."[5] Those found with clinical signs of the disease were only to be isolated if yielding positive bacteriological examination results whereas "Native Full Bloods" were to be isolated even if such results proved negative. In the case of suspects (those without clinical or bacteriological evidence of the disease), "Native Full Bloods" were to be detained until a definite diagnosis could be made while corresponding Europeans were to be discharged and kept under medical surveillance.[6]

The most significant changes for European patients were implemented in the late 1950s when, after taking study tours to Hong Kong and the United States, the Queensland Director-General of Health, Abraham Fryberg, relaxed requirements "for the release of white patients from strict isolation."[7] The number of consecutive negative smear results required for discharge from Queensland's Peel Island Leprosarium, where most European patients in Australia were detained, was reduced from twelve to three. The following year, those who had not already been discharged under the new policy were transferred to Brisbane's Princess Alexandria Hospital and the leprosarium was closed.[8] Proportionately large discharges also occurred at lazarets in Perth and Sydney, leaving only residents who had become dependent on the institutions due to disabilities. The net effect was to reduce the total number of European patients in isolation from seventy-six in 1950 to nineteen in 1960, by which time Indigenous patients accounted for 94% of the total population in isolation in Australia.[9]

Strict isolation requirements for Indigenous people arose partly from the perception by the middle of the 1950s, that leprosy in the European population was petering out while increasing and spreading out among Indigenous groups. Having been the only region where the disease had been endemic in both races, Queensland was enjoying decreasing notifications overall, even when active case-finding operatives were carried out. Conversely, medical surveys from the 1950s to the mid-1960s revealed significant numbers of untreated Indigenous sufferers in the Northern Territory and northern Western Australia and, furthermore, showed that the disease was infiltrating previously unaffected regions. Between the early 1940s and the mid-1950s in the Northern Territory, the course of the disease had fanned out from the extreme north and north-west, around Pine Creek and the Tiwi Islands, to East Arnhem Land in the east, south to Tennant Creek, and west to the pastoral stations close to the Western Australia border. In Western Australia, the centre of activity had shifted from the Western Kimberley near Broome and Beagle Bay to include the north-east, the far north of the state and down along the eastern border, contiguous with the Northern Territory. New notifications between the early 1950s and late 1960s continued to come from a much wider area than from the concentrated pockets identified prior to the Second World War, as different Indigenous groups gradually became infected.[10] A.J. Metcalfe, holding the twins posts of Commonwealth Director-General of Health and NHMRC Chairman between 1946 and 1960, had in 1953 publicly declared that "leprosy was the worst medical problem in Northern Australia."[11] Consequently, official leprosy policy, while remaining vigilant over other areas and with respect to other races, turned predominantly to the management of Indigenous populations in this endemic region comprising the expansive confluent areas of northern Western Australia and northern Northern Territory.

Racially disparate leprosy policies were to some extent based on assumptions held by some influential health bureaucrats that Indigenous people's was conducive to the spread of disease. One example put forward by senior medical administrators in the 1950s was a predilection for moving around from place to place. Reporting on the epidemiology of the disease in the Northern Territory in 1952, Director of Health, A.H. Humphry, attributed its spread to the wandering at large of Channel Island patients after being released during the bombing of Darwin in 1942. Patients in Queensland, on the other hand, had remained secured during this period.[12] Some months later, Fryberg told a conference, "…in all Queensland there were very few wandering natives, and probably for that reason there was a lower incidence of leprosy in Queensland than in the Northern Territory."[13] One longstanding fear, persisting from the interwar period, was that Indigenous people would take leprosy south beyond the twentieth degree of latitude and threaten settled European populations. In 1941, Western Australia legislated to forbid all Indigenous people to pass this point, known as the 'Leper Line', without a permit stating special reasons, such as for medical purposes or work. The legislation remained in place, with some expansion of permits, until 1963.[14] In the Northern Territory in 1962, Health Director Ian Byrne considered the prospect of leprosy being spread south to Central Australia "a disaster of appalling magnitude" and he urged the Welfare Branch to "ensure that there is no intercourse of any kind between natives of the leprosy free Centre and those of leprosy endemic North."[15]

The NHMRC criteria for leprosarium isolation and discharge were based on a presumed medical 'knowledge' about Indigenous people and the conditions in which they lived. Any patients who had been successfully treated with the sulphones were not really cured; their disease had merely arrested and was liable to reactivate if the drugs were not taken regularly and indefinitely, or if diet and hygiene were inadequate. To be discharged home, patients had to have a fixed address, to continue their medication to avoid relapse and to attend regular medical examinations. They also needed "separate accommodation and utensils, an adequate diet and no domiciliary contact with children."[16] These latter elements were precisely what Indigenous people lacked, according to medical administrators, such as Humphry. When justifying the application of the NHMRC recommendations to Northern Territory Indigenous people, he implied that these deficiencies were due to their own natural tendencies: "his standard of hygiene is poor, he will not sleep apart, nor can he restrain his intense fondness for children. He does not understand the word 'infectivity'"[17] These attributes, or the idea of them, cost Indigenous leprosy patients dearly. From the late 1950s, they were detained for three to four years in a leprosarium whereas Europeans, under the relaxed rules, spent just a few months in a hospital.

As the author has argued elsewhere, the focus on the perceived failings of Indigenous people regarding their health and hygiene practices masked, to some degree, the structural factors militating against their discharge home. In reality, poor diet and hygiene, overcrowded and substandard housing, and the lack of health services in some missions, government settlements and other Indigenous communities were to blame. Medical administrators acknowledged that the absence of medical clinics and nurses in some patients' home areas was the reason they refused to allow patients to be discharged, or they arranged for them to be sent elsewhere.[18]

To a large extent, the Sisters kept control of these factors in the leprosarium. Moreover, if patients required special care such as for ulcers or disabilities, they were retained in the leprosarium until it was safe for them to live independently. Health authorities continued to support the original 1950 NHMRC resolution stating that discharge from isolation could only occur if the patient was able to maintain a minimum living standard, a fixed address, and proximity to medical supervision. There was much less hope for Indigenous people to be discharged as "it will be apparent that Europeans in general may be expected to be more consistent in satisfying these requirements than will the native races."[19] When Derby leprosarium reported high rates of readmissions due to relapses more than ten years after treatment with the sulphones had begun, Byrne vowed to maintain "tight leprosy control."[20]

North-western Western Australia took many years longer than the Northern Territory to incorporate three important components of leprosy care: Indigenous health assistants (late 1970s), public health survey nurses (late 1960s) and injectable long-acting sulphones (mid-1970s). All of these elements facilitated outpatient treatment and therefore allowed remotely located Indigenous people to continue treatment while working and living normally. Without them, patients had to be retained at

Derby leprosarium longer than necessary. It was only on the condition that adequate medical surveillance could continue after release from the leprosarium that the NHMRC relaxed its stringent discharge policies in 1967.[21] Furthermore, a Commonwealth parliamentary inquiry into Indigenous health in 1979 concluded that these measures were responsible for the significant decline in new leprosy notifications in the Northern Territory between 1967 and 1977.[22]

Indigenous patients' prospects for resuming normal lives in the 1950s were further dashed by the failure of governments to institute corrective surgery and rehabilitation services. The informal occupational therapy given by the Sisters did not take the place of trained therapists with the ability to teach practical and specific work skills to patients that could be realistically used in the current demands of the outside world. In 1953, the Relatives and Friends Association (RFA) inquired as to the eligibility of recovering leprosy patients for the Commonwealth government rehabilitation scheme established in 1948 for invalid pensioners, as part of its welfare reforms. The Director of the Department of Social Services stated that it would not be productive to include them since public prejudice made their re-establishment in the community "almost hopeless" but that "the problem is not a big one because the number of whites suffering from Hansen's Disease is small."[23] However, in 1956, the Director-General, newly enlightened by medical wisdom and citing the psychological benefits of rehabilitation and the low infectivity of the disease, allowed only white patients to join their programme, noting with almost tangible relief that "very few cases are likely to arise" and probably "only in Queensland."[24]

Agitation for Patients' Rights at East Arm

In the 1960s, some religious leprosarium staff began agitating strongly for better conditions and outcomes for the patients. The most prominent advocate was Mother Marion Whelan OLSH, the matron and religious superior at East Arm Leprosarium between 1959 and 1966. She and John Hargrave, the medical superintendent, fought government departments to lessen harsh regulations and systemic inequities that disadvantaged their patients and families. They were critical especially of the tough Territory policies in the early 1960s for patient discharge contained in the NHMRC's recommendations. Hargrave preferred patients to stay in the leprosarium for the minimum period required. He believed that prolonged isolation was unnecessary and inhumane, and, further, deterred sufferers from volunteering for treatment. In 1961, Byrne, on behalf of the Commonwealth Director-General of Health, issued an order that any patient who had a single positive bacterial test result was to remain indefinitely in isolation. Hargrave was warned not to discharge any patients without his personal permission.[25] Abouttwo years later, Byrne's Acting Director complained to the Director-General that Hargrave was continuing to disregard the NHMRC criteria and that "his views on the subject are to say the least, radical, but are in my opinion alarming".[26]

Mother Marion also opposed the lengthy detention of patients who were physically well and who were aware of their eligibility for discharge. She felt that this practice led to escalating violence and anti-social behaviour among the patients. In 1962, she wrote to Byrne, expressing her strong disapproval of the departmental policies:

> Since we have, by maintaining a somewhat outmoded and unenlightened policy on leprosy control, contributed to a number of our present problems, we will probably have to put up with them to some degree. One wonders how many lives have to be wrecked before someone will consider it 'worthwhile' to consider a more rational, more up to date approach, taking into consideration the vast advances in leprosy treatment which have been made over the past twenty years. In the days when leprosy was almost inevitably a life sentence many of these regulations may, though regrettable, have been necessary.[27]

For Mother Marion, other suggested measures, such as increased surveillance and security, including the deployment of round-the-clock security guards, locked gates and the use of a detention cell, were never going to solve the problems. Rather, a more understanding approach was required, given the psychological problems induced by the patients' incarceration. She suggested to Byrne that the patients be permitted "short periods of leave" because "this in itself would provide a safety valve for many of the tensions which must lead to some type of outburst in most individuals."[28]

As Mother Marion tried to impress on Byrne, the patients' awareness of the anomalies of their situation compared with leprosy patients elsewhere only intensified their misery and added further to the possibility of anti-social behaviour. "They would have to be very dull not to know they were getting better and have only to read *Post* or *Time* to get a fairly accurate idea of modern trends in leprosy policy."[29]

Byrne was determined to see that his department's policies were implemented, no matter what the staff thought,

> We maintain and enforce our present Departmental policy in full and even render it more stringent and apply it more vigorously...That we commence now a drive to isolate all lepers in the leprosarium...That we be prepared...to lose the services of the Sisters who now staff the leprosarium and to lose the services of Dr Hargrave and prepare to replace them if they find themselves unable to accept our policy and all it implies.[30]

Another anomaly Mother Marion raised was the inequitable distribution of Commonwealth social security payments. Although, in 1959, the Commonwealth government extended old age and invalid pensions to Indigenous people (other than the "nomadic or primitive"), in the case of leprosarium patients, most of the money was retained by State and Territory governments. European patients, however, were paid their full pensions directly. This practice also occurred on some settlements, missions and pastoral properties, although the amounts withheld varied.[31] At East Arm in 1961, of the £10.10s total fortnightly pension, £6.16 was deposited into the health department's revenue account to pay for patients' treatment and upkeep; £2.14 into a trust account with the Commonwealth Bank; and £1 given directly to the patient as "pocket money."[32] The cost of maintaining one patient at this time was £6 per week.[33]

The racial disparity in the leprosarium can be explained, largely, by the same preconceptions operating on missions and settlements, about Indigenous people's use of cash. Even if they were legally entitled to pensions or wages, they were not considered as entirely deserving of them by mission heads and government officers, who expected the money would be spent unwisely. The Commonwealth Director-General took this much further in his nightmarish visions of cashed-up patients at East Arm:

> It is to be confidently expected that payment of some 30/- weekly to natives detained under treatment for leprosy at East Arm Settlement will make the Institution completely unmanageable. Gambling, indulgence in alcohol, prostitution and hire car traffic between the settlement and nearby Darwin would very seriously impair the discipline in an Institution at present largely managed by Sisters of a religious order...[34]

In other words, money, if plentiful, could undo all that the Sisters had achieved in establishing an orderly and morally wholesome domain (Fig. 10.1).

But there were more reasons against giving patients the full amount of their pension, as the Director-General outlined in 1961. They might cease doing their chores, depriving them of the inherent benefits of labour: discipline, community living, mental and physical health, and rehabilitation.[35] Furthermore, he felt that the patients should contribute to the cost of their upkeep. After all, they were given "free medical service…quartered, fed and supplied with some clothing"[36] Here then he was suggesting a contractual obligation between the patients and the health department to which the former had never consented, and which was not considered for European patients. What was truly disturbing to the Commonwealth Health Department were the imagined consequences of paying about £12,000 accrued since the pension had been extended, all at once to 100 patients, "whose needs are relatively simple…[and]

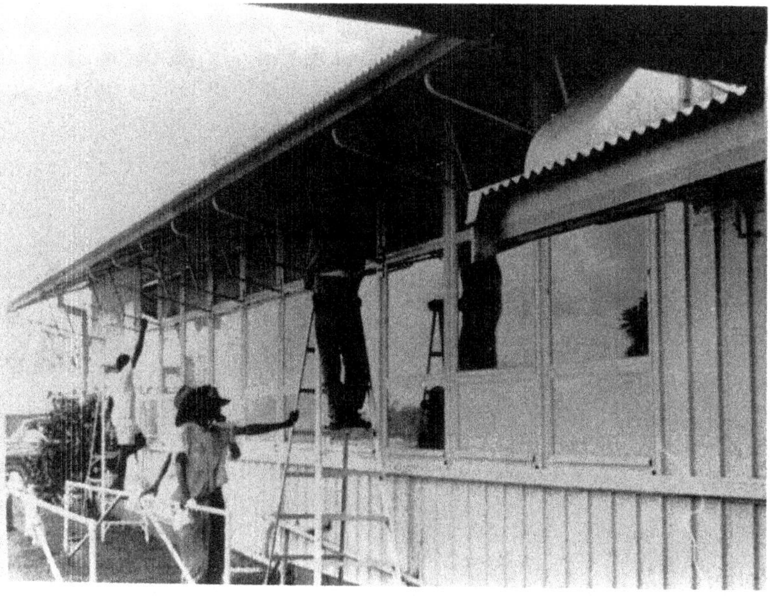

Fig. 10.1 'Male patients doing building repairs 1961' [East Arm Leprosarium] (Charles Darwin University Nursing Museum)

might well result in large scale absconding with an inevitable crop of civil offences in Darwin Township."[37]

In her protest in 1963 to William Refshauge, the Commonwealth Director-General of Health, Mother Marion wrote, "...quite a number of the native patients are unhappy about not receiving anything like the amount received by European and part-coloured patients. It is difficult to explain this on any other grounds than racial discrimination."[38] Such was the anxiety of the bureaucracy about allowing Indigenous people financial autonomy that, at first, the complaints were ignored, then reactivated after further prompting from Hargrave, then passed along from one department to another then subjected to inquiry at a joint meeting of the Commonwealth departments of Social Services, Health and the Treasury in February 1965. The conference decided to defer the matter while considering whether to classify the leprosarium as a "benevolent institution" in which case pension funds could be withheld from residents anyway.[39]

Mother Marion and Hargrave also suggested in 1963 that the accumulated funds held back from Indigenous people's pensions might be used for amenities, such as a swimming pool. "... it would be a way of reducing our behaviour problems...One can often see quite clearly that they arise from sheer boredom."[40] Initially, the health department refused to give permission on the grounds that it could assist the spread of leprosy. However, eventually the pool was built.[41]

Despite her contestation of decisions made by the Health Department, Mother Marion maintained a public façade of solidarity with government authorities. In September 1962, she became "seriously concerned for the safety of the Sisters" when some patients, after illicitly gaining access to alcohol, committed violent assaults on others.[42] The perpetrators had begun paying nocturnal visits to the convent and the Sisters had been trying to protect the young women who worked at the convent from them. "But who is to protect the protectors?" Mother Marion asked Byrne.[43] In November, she was asked to refute a statement made by a member of parliament that the Sisters were "in real fear of being attacked by patients."[44] In response, she issued a statement denying his claim and asserting that the Sisters were satisfied with the security at East Arm. While she admitted that there were "some behaviour problems" among the patients, she did not reveal the view expressed to Byrne—that the Department's policies were responsible—but ascribed them to "a community which is so circumscribed and composed of so many different elements" and "people outside the leprosarium who continue to make intoxicants available to patients."[45]

Agitation at Derby and Fantome Island

By 1965, many of the battles had been won, and the Commonwealth government was promoting East Arm as a modern and enlightened facility in the capable hands of Hargrave and Mother Marion. It was a "specialised reconstructive unit, the only one of its kind in Australia," and in which "isolation need only be applied to patients who are passing through a period of infectivity."[46] Therequirement by the NHMRC for medical surveillance of discharged patients had been possible in the Northern Territory due to increased field staff, including survey sisters and Indigenous health assistants, since the late 1950s. In the leprosarium in the late 1960s, the religious nursing Sisters applied intensive occupational therapy sessions, and outsourced services trained the patients in trades and other industries through which they could earn money. By 1970, patients were making jewellery, printing Christmas cards, and growing seedlings for forest plantations. As a result, more and more specialist lay staff became involved in the patients' care and training.[47] In 1971, East Arm finally secured the services of a full-time physiotherapist.[48]

Before considering how religious staff at the other two leprosaria dealt with unsatisfactory conditions, it is necessary to explore how these institutions developed in relation to East Arm. At Fantome Island, nothing like the same advances occurred. Neither surgical programmes nor formal rehabilitation programmes were ever introduced. Treatment was limited as "a doctor who has little knowledge of leprosy now visits Fantome Island once a week and the Sisters cannot be asked to administer any treatment needing fairly close medical supervision."[49] In 1953, the Sisters rejected the offer of the Australian Red Cross Society to introduce handcrafts lessons. At this time, its workers regularly attended Peel Island where they taught the patients to make items such as bags, belts, shoes, and baskets from leather, plastic, and cane.[50] After being contacted by the RFA, Townsville Red Cross Secretary, Mrs Mousally, visited Fantome Island with a view to doing the same, reporting later that the Superior, Mother St Nérée, had said the programme was not possible due to the requirement for extra staff to supervise the "costly" materials. And, further, "that it was already difficult to make the patients do all that was required of them such as keeping themselves and their huts clean..." It is quite evident that Mother St Nérée viewed the proposal as a poor reflection on the Sisters' own efforts, and saw it as an unwelcome interference. Undoubtedly, the patients' "lavish display of embroidery" and the "women… busy knitting" noted by an admiring Mrs Mousally were ploys to convince her of the futility of her mission.[51]

There is very little evidence to indicate that the Queensland government was interested in improving therapeutics and social conditions for the patients, presumably because, from the late 1950s, with so few in detention and no lingering threat from the disease apparent, leprosy and its sufferers slipped from the health department's radar. In 1965, it began considering closing the leprosarium due to low patient numbers. Medical officer, Morgan Gabriel, advised relocating the patients to the Princess Alexandria hospital in Brisbane, where European leprosy patients were accommodated in a special unit. The Indigenous patients could then receive the same treatment, such as regular expert medical attention and rehabilitation services. He added that, like the European patients, they could control their own money. Gabriel also recommended applying the same isolation and release criteria to Indigenous patients as were in place for European patients. "We would be able to say that there was absolutely no discrimination between white and coloured patients with Hansen's Disease."[52] Hisadvice was not taken.

The government failed to maintain living conditions to a decent standard on Fantome Island. By the middle of the 1960s, the housing was run down, facilities outdated, and essential services primitive. Father Maurice Malone OFM, the resident chaplain, bombarded Patrick Killoran, Director of the Queensland Department of Aboriginal and Island Affairs (DAIA) with long letters criticising the conditions. His list of grievances included the water shortage, malfunctioning refrigeration and the unreliable D.C. electricity supply. Malone's campaign was on behalf of the entire but small Fantome Island community, but he especially railed at the trials of the Sisters who had a "never complain attitude."[53] He had little support from the Townsville bishop, Leonard Faulkner. Writing for the *Townsville Catholic News* after a visit to the island in this period, he mentioned the poor conditions, but, far from expressing his disapproval, took the attitude of his predecessors in extolling Christian forbearance: "The phone is a chancy affair and there is no A.C. electricity. The Sisters very seldom leave the Island. Yet they are happy that they are serving God and His 'little ones' there."[54]

A petition sent by patients to the Queensland Director-General of Health in 1969 echoed Malone's complaints. The patients, many of whom had disabilities, described how, to cook meals, they had to collect and cut wood for the stove. The buildings were rusted, leaking, and "riddled with white ants."[55] Killoran dismissed the petition, claiming it was engineered by Father Malone, who was suffering from ill-health. The solution for Killoran, as with his predecessors, was to remove the troublemaker, and so Malone's superiors withdrew him from the island.[56] However, the complaints were backed by Sister Ubald, who had become matron the previous year. Informed by the health department of the patients' petition, she confirmed the poor state of the buildings and wrote that "we were left for five days without water... We were able to collect water in a bucket, drop by drop, from what was left at the bottom of the tanks. This is the reason why the patients were so agitated."[57] As a result, some improvements to buildings and facilities followed.

In 1971, an inspection by the medical superintendent of Townsville Hospital, David Bowler, revealed the severe shortcomings of Fantome Island as a residential treatment centre for leprosy. Bowler's criticisms were aimed at the lack of recreational and occupational therapy services.

> As members of society their position is tragic, and it is a reflection on the Administration not on the provision of medical care, which is easy, but in the complete lack of appreciation of the social problems of Hansen's disease, and the lack of any provision whatever to enable these outcasts to lead productive lives.[58]

Despite the surgical programme at Derby following close on the heels of that at East Arm, the former never evolved to be able to provide the advanced level of care provided by John Hargrave and his team. This difference does not reflect any less enthusiasm or competence on the part of the doctors and Sisters at Derby, but more a reluctance of the Western Australian government to provide the necessary funds and support. Derby had comparable numbers of patients with those at East Arm, but medical officers in the 1960s and 1970s at the former had to combine their leprosarium work with a range of other health department duties. The leprosarium had poor theatre equipment and other hospital facilities, could not provide patients with surgical boots and callipers, and had insufficient professional physiotherapy services, meaning that reconstructive surgery was either performed under difficult conditions or deferred (Fig. 10.2).[59]

Between 1967 and 1968, Derby medical officer, John Elphinstone, who also had charge of the leprosarium, petitioned the Commissioner of Public Health and the Minister of Health to increase field nursing staff and update treatment. As with Morgan Gabriel in Queensland, he was critical of the racial inequities in health care and the isolation policy.

> The hardship of prolonged segregation which inadequate field staff inevitably imposes on leprosy patients sometimes for years longer than should be necessary is something for which the Public Health Dept of WA

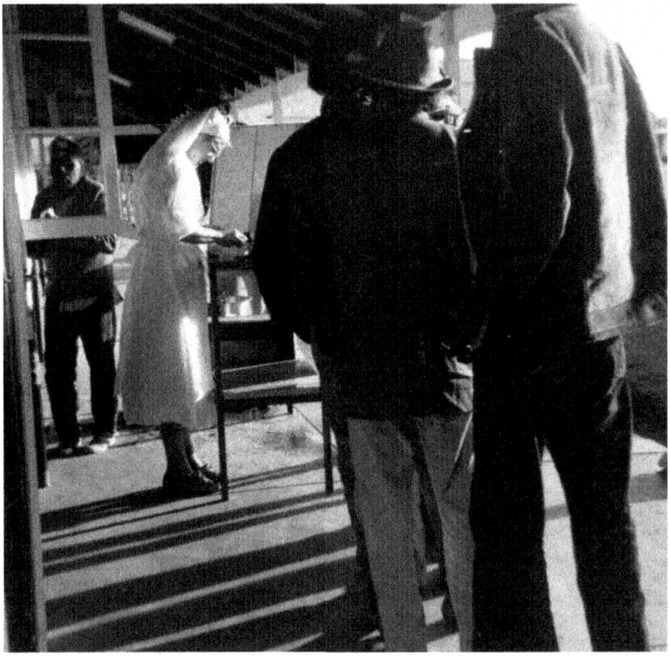

Fig. 10.2 Patients lined up for medicine given out by Sister Camille, Derby Leprosarium 1960s (SSJG Heritage Centre Broome)

> must take full responsibility. One wonders whether its attitude of indifference would be the same if the majority of leprosy patients were not Aboriginal or part-Aboriginal.[60]

Although having been ten years in his post, these complaints led to his demotion in 1968 to a hospital position in the state's capital city, Perth.[61] He subsequently took these issues to federal parliament and the press, comparing the more generous staffing and resources in the Northern Territory with those in Western Australia, and calling for Commonwealth control over Western Australia's leprosy management. Shortly after his departure, the Public Health Commissioner of Western Australia, W.S. Davidson, who had clashed with Elphinstone over the latter's criticisms, announced a $500,000 plan for leprosy policy reforms. The leprosarium was to be updated with a new hospital and patient accommodation, and public health nurses and clerical staff would be increased.[62] Before leaving the north, Elphinstone wrote to Mother Alphonsus to thank her "for all the help and encouragement you have given me over many years, and hope that the future holds brighter prospects for our work."[63] But almost certainly the Sisters' support did not extend to backing Elphinstone's recent public campaign. One of his supporters, health department nurse, Marie Osborn, complained to a politician who had taken up Elphinstone's case, of a "conspiratorial web of silence" that included "the Nursing Staff, all two of them of a religious order, and therefore silent."[64]

If the Derby Sisters did not call the government to account publicly, there is evidence, by 1970, of their private pressure for changes. In her visitation report of that year, the Provincial Superior described the room where operations were performed as "appalling in this day and age" and said that the Sisters "could do so much more" for the patients if new hospital and administration blocks and an operating theatre were installed. "There is a limit to human endurance and I regret to say that unless some steps are taken to improve the set up here, the sisters will have to be withdrawn."[65] By the middle of 1973, the Sisters remained on staff, despite the works not being undertaken. "...The efforts of the sisters to secure a new hospital block have been unavailing and government policy regarding the hospitals causes anxiety and concern."[66] Eventually, the works were completed, but by that time, patient numbers had decreased to the point that they were hardly necessary.[67]

In trying to account for the failure of the two state governments to properly fund leprosy treatment in this period, it is important to remember that even in the 1930s, significant disease management initiatives were only ever enacted after pressure from interest groups and with financial subsidies from the Commonwealth government, either directly or through the NHMRC for field surveys and setting up the two leprosaria. The treatment, undertaken almost entirely by the religious nursing Sisters using cheap medication, was inexpensive for state health departments. To be brought up to the standard employed in the Northern Territory in the 1960s, including outpatient and inpatient care, much higher expenditure was required, with the necessity of providing improved health services to Indigenous communities as part of leprosy surveillance programmes. Health historians Margaret-Ann Franklin and Isobel White argue that until the 1970s "the states tended to ignore the special health needs of Aborigines" and even then only undertook some improvements to health services with finance from the new Commonwealth Office of Aboriginal Affairs.[68] This time, neither the state of Indigenous health nor the threat of the disease to public health was sufficient to invoke the groundswell of criticism that had propelled the Commonwealth's interwar leprosy campaign into Queensland and Western Australia. From the NHMRC in 1967 and 1973 came tactful allusions to the disparate policies across the states and territories with the statement that to avoid undesirable long-term isolation of patients, the states should provide appropriate facilities, but there was no attempt to compel standardisation.[69]

Some contrasts can be drawn between the kinds of protests mounted by the Sisters working in the state leprosaria, and those in the Commonwealth leprosarium at East Arm. At the former, the Western Australian and Queensland governments failed to update medical equipment and basic services, and these inadequacies were the basis of complaints by the Sisters, doctors, and the Fantome Island priest. However, Mother Marion's grievances were related to patients' rights—to their freedom from isolation, their mental well-being in the leprosarium, and their right to their own money. East Arm was twenty years newer than the other institutions and continued to be updated, so staff did not have cause for complaints in this regard. Mother Marion was also unafraid to directly criticise government officers for their policies and to pressure them individually for change. Sisters in the state institutions seemed more supportive of the status quo, but this is hardly surprising considering their ages and the periods they had worked in the leprosaria. Many of the Fantome Island Sisters who arrived in the 1940s were still on staff twenty to thirty years later and some were in their sixties and seventies. At Derby in the late 1960s, the same can be said for Mother Alphonsus who had been at the leprosarium since 1940 and, although no longer a Superior, continued to hold authority. These Sisters were of a generation of women religious who were more accepting of privation and, moreover, having lived in the leprosaria from early days, knew little else but humble conditions. The leprosarium was their life's work, therefore they were less likely to risk losing it through upsetting the authorities. They were also to some degree more insulated from the broader social changes of the 1950s and 1960s. In contrast, the East Arm Sisters were rotated regularly to work on the missions, in line with their order's policy. Mother Marion, therefore, did not form a long association with East Arm, and being relatively young, was open to new developments outside the leprosarium due to greater exposure to doctors, welfare officers and others (Fig. 10.3).

Despite the potential to profoundly improve the lives of Indigenous people with leprosy, the medical advances that emerged after the late 1940s proved disappointing for many. Therapeutic changes were introduced slowly and incompletely. East Arm leprosarium was the only institution to provide high standard comprehensive treatment and rehabilitation services, due to committed religious and lay staff and a concerted effort by the Commonwealth government. At the state-controlled institutions of Fantome Island and Derby, these services were either never incorporated, or only slowly and partially provided.

Indigenous sufferers were also disadvantaged by the persistence of stringent isolation practices that continued until at least the early 1970s in Western Australia and Queensland and until the middle of the 1960s in the Northern Territory, despite international recommendations for their relaxation in 1950 after demonstrated success with sulphone therapy and the more liberal conditions for European sufferers in Australia since the late 1950s. Indigenous sufferers in non-infectious stages of leprosy were prevented from remaining in, or returning to, their home communities if they could not support themselves, could not access nursing services or were disabled.

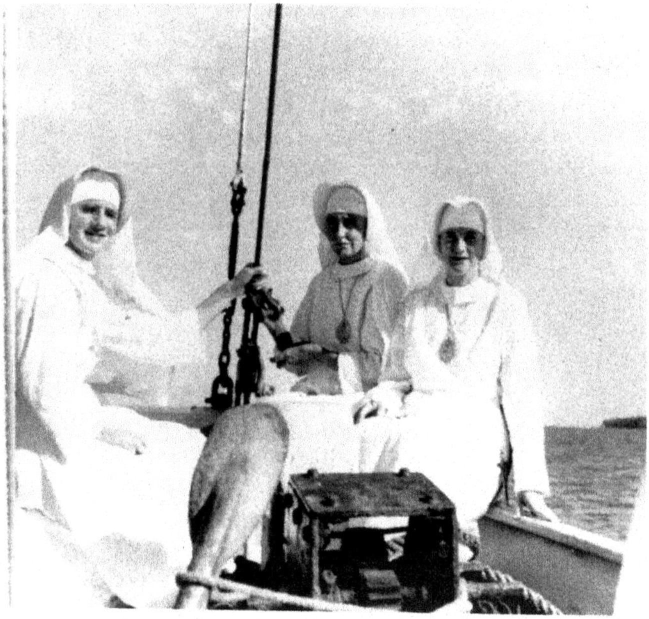

Fig. 10.3 'Catholic Nursing sisters from East Arm leprosarium 1961' (Charles Darwin University Nursing Museum)

In the Northern Territory, the ideals of the assimilation policy were used in a positive sense, to justify and further the more rapid pace and extent of therapeutic developments, and the ultimate tempering of the isolation policy, all of which were well in progress by the middle of the 1960s. Here, along with their clinical work, doctors and Catholic Sisters fought against systemic inequities that retarded patients' access to a decent standard of health and welfare, and the Commonwealth government, concerned with its international image, ultimately fostered their efforts. Avenues for corresponding developments in northern Western Australia and northern Queensland were never opened to the same extent, in spite of pressure from doctors and some religious staff. Nonetheless, due to the assiduous efforts of medical and nursing staff at Derby and Fantome Island, hundreds of Indigenous sufferers were restored to health and their lives saved.

Notes

1. World Health Organisation (WHO) Expert Committee on Leprosy. 1953. *WHO Expert Committee on Leprosy: First Report*. Geneva: WHO, 9, 4–6.
2. Ibid., 9.
3. Ibid.
4. Report of the National Health and Medical Research Council (NHMRC) Committee on Tropical Physiology and Hygiene, November 2, 1950, 2. (A1658, 258/1/1 PART 1), National Archives of Australia (NAA); NHMRC. 1958. 'Leprosy and Its Management', in Commonwealth Department of Health, 1958. *Health*. Canberra: The Department, March, 21.
5. Report of the NHMRC Committee, 3.
6. Ibid., 2–4.
7. Fryberg, Abraham. 1960. 'Hansen's Disease in the White Population,' Queensland Health and Medical Services Branch, *Annual Report on the Health and Medical Services of the State of Queensland 1958–1959*. Brisbane: The State, 20.
8. Ibid.
9. Commonwealth Bureau of Census and Statistics. 1953. *Official Year Book of the Commonwealth of Australia No. 39, 1953*. Canberra: Commonwealth Government Printer, 303; Commonwealth Bureau of Census and Statistics. 1961. *Official Year Book of the Commonwealth of Australia Book No. 47*, Canberra: Commonwealth Government Printer, 685.
10. Hargrave, J.C. 1975. 'Leprosy in the Northern Territory of Australia: With Particular Reference to the Aborigines of Arnhem Land and the Arid Regions of the Northern Territory'. M.D. Diss., University of Sydney, 39–40, 45–60, 298; Davidson, W.S. 1978. *Havens of Refuge: A History of Leprosy in Western Australia*, Perth: University of Western Australia Press for the Public Health Department, 138–145; Parliament of the Commonwealth of Australia. 1955–1962. *Report(s) on the Administration of the Northern Territory for the Years 1955–1962*. Canberra: Government of the Commonwealth of Australia.
11. 'Leprosy Increases Hold on Natives'. *The West Australian*. February 18, 1953,1.
12. Humphry, A.H. 1952. 'Leprosy Among Full-Blooded Aborigines.' *The Medical Journal of Australia (MJA)*. April 1, 570.
13. 'The Epidemiology and Control of Leprosy'. *MJA*. October 18, 1952, 568.
14. Davidson, *Havens of Refuge*, 104–105.
15. Byrne, Ian (Northern Territory Director of Health) to Director of Welfare, August 30, 1962 (F1, 1959/975), NAA.
16. Report of the NHMRC Committee, 3.

17. Humphry, 'Leprosy Among Full-Blooded Aborigines', 572.
18. Robson, Charmaine. 2016. 'Ending Isolation? Leprosy, Welfare and Indigenous Australians 1950–86.' Aboriginal History 40, 65–88.
19. Report of the NHMRC Committee, 1.
20. Byrne to Director of Welfare, August 30, 1962 (F1, 1959/975), NAA.
21. 'Leprosy Control in Australia'. *MJA*. December 30, 1967, 1209.
22. Western Australia Public Health Department (WAPHD). 1968. *Report of the Commissioner of Public Health*. Perth, Western Australia: Department of Public Health, 60, 66–67; WAPHD. 1973. *Report*, 63; WAPHD. 1980. *Report*, 176; Parliament of the Commonwealth of Australia. 1979. *Standing Committee on Aboriginal Affairs, Aboriginal Health*, Canberra: Australian Government Printing Service, 22, 83.
23. Director, Department of Social Services (DSS) to Director-General, July 29, 1953 (A886, C174), NAA.
24. Director-General, DSS to Minister for Social Services, May 4, 1956 (A886, C174), NAA.
25. Byrne to Hargrave, John, August 22, 1961 (A1658, 756/11/1 PART 2), NAA.
26. Langsford, Stephen to Refshauge, William, January 15, 1963 (A1658, 756/11/1 PART 2), NAA.
27. Whelan, Sr Marion to Byrne, September 25, 1962 (A1658, 756/11/1 PART 2), NAA.
28. Ibid.
29. Ibid.
30. Byrne quoted in Kettle, Ellen. 1991. *Health Services in the Northern Territory: A History 1824–1970*, Volume two. Darwin: North Australia Research Unit, 52.
31. Kidd, Rosalind. 2006. *Trustees on Trial: Recovering the Stolen Wages*. Canberra: Aboriginal Studies Press, 96–7.
32. Byrne to Refshauge, October 13, 1961 (A1658, 756/11/1 PART 2), NAA.
33. Refshauge to Director-General, DSS, July 13, 1961 (A1658, 756/11/1 PART 2), NAA.
34. Refshauge to Secretary, Deparment of Territories, March 1959 (A884, A55 PART II), NAA.
35. Refshauge to Director-General, DSS, July 13, 1961 (A1658, 756/11/1 PART 2), NAA.
36. Ibid.
37. Ibid.
38. Mother Marion to Refshauge, November 18, 1963 (A1658, 756/11/1 PART 2), NAA.
39. 'Notes on Conference at Treasury on 19th February 1965' (A1658, 756/11/1 PART 2), NAA.

40. Mother Marion to Refshauge, November 18, 1963 (A1658, 756/11/1 PART 2), NAA.
41. Kettle, *Health Services*, 53.
42. Mother Marion to Byrne, September 25, 1962 (A1658, 756/11/1 PART 2), NAA.
43. Ibid.
44. Byrne to Assistant Administrator, November 9, 1962 (A1658, 756/11/1 PART 2), NAA.
45. Mother Marion, Statement, November 9, 1962 (A1658, 756/11/1 PART 2), NAA.
46. Hargrave, John and Mother Marion. 1965. 'New Approach to Old Problem'. *Australian Territories* 5(6), 34- 35.
47. 'Report of meeting of the East Arm Rehabilitation Committee, 5 October 1970'. (F1, 1969/2678), NAA.
48. Kettle, *Health Services,* 53.
49. Gabriel, Morgan to Director-General, Queensland Department of Health and Medical Services (DHMS), September 17, 1965. (Director of Native Affairs Office, 3A/157, Correspondence, Aboriginal and Torres Strait Islander, ID ITM505023), Queensland State Archives (QSA).
50. Queensland Health and Medical Services Branch, *Annual Report 1955*, 16–17.
51. Mousally to Assistant Director, Queensland Department of Native Affairs, May 9, 1952. (3A/157, ITM505023), QSA.
52. Gabriel to DHMS, September 17, 1965 (3A/157, ITM505023), QSA.
53. Malone, Father Maurice OFM to Killoran, Patrick, January 19, 1967 (3A/157, ITM505023), QSA.
54. Faulkner, Bishop L. 1968. 'Visitation of Fantome Island Leprosarium', *Townsville Catholic News*. October, 2.
55. Fantome Island Patients. 1969. Petition addressed to DHMS. (3A/157, ITM505023), QSA.
56. Ibid.; Killoran to DHMS, March 13, 1969 (3A/157, ITM505023), QSA.
57. Bellamare, Sr Ubald to DHMS, March 4, 1969 (3A/157, ITM505023), QSA.
58. Bowler, David. 'Report for Public Hospitals Board, 18 January 1971. (Item ID 505,023), QSA.
59. WAPHD. 1968, *Report*, 57; WAPHD. 1969, *Report*, 49; WAPHD. 1971, *Report*, 54.
60. Elphinstone, J.J. c.1968. 'Medieval Lazaret Policy in Western Australia'. (MN 1454, Papers of J.J. Elphinstone, ACC 4585A/4), Battye Library.
61. Elphinstone to Daly, Sr Alphonsus, May 25, 1968. (MN 1454, Papers of J.J. Elphinstone, ACC 4585A/4), Battye Library.
62. 'News', *The West Australian*, June 3, 1968.
63. Elphinstone to Sr Alphonsus, May 25, 1968.

64. Osborn, Marie to Tonkin, J.T. MLA, September 6, 1969 (MN 1454, Papers of J.J. Elphinstone, ACC 4585A/4), Battye Library.
65. Naturtas, Sister M. 1970. 'Extracts from Visitation of Provincials and Generals 1937–1976'. June 23, 1970. (2.621), Sisters of St John of God Archives, Broome (SSJGB).
66. Justinian, Sr M. 'Extracts from Visitation of Provincials and Generals 1937–1976.' June 11, 1973. (2.621), SSJGB.
67. 'Jottings of Sisters A. Moroney, C. Poidevin, N. Ryan, F. Dunne, D. Spargo, and the Internet. To be delivered at the St John of God Leaders of the Mission National Meeting by Sr F. Dunne on 8 March 2002. (2.21Y), SSJGB.
68. Franklin, Margaret-Ann and Isobel White. 1991. 'The History and Politics of Aboriginal Health'. In *The Health of Aboriginal Australia*, ed. Janice Reid and Peggy Trompf. Marrickville: Harcourt Brace & Company, 26–27.
69. 'Leprosy Control in Australia', 1209–1210; NHMRC, 1973. 'Appendix XXXVII: Leprosy Control in Australia', in *NHMRC: Report of the Seventy-seventh Session*. Canberra: AGPS, 198.

CHAPTER 11

Recollections, Connections and Conclusions

Recollections and Connections

One by one the leprosaria closed as the incidence of the disease in their different regions declined and methods of local control improved. Fantome Island, in 1973, was the first, in accordance with Queensland's early changing epidemiological pattern. East Arm followed in 1982 and Derby, Australia's last leprosarium to close, four years later, spelling the end of perhaps the most racially based public health policy. Leprosy cases were thereafter treated either in regional hospitals or in outpatient community settings. At last, Indigenous people need not have feared that diagnosis would lead to removal from their homes or long-term confinement in special institutions.

At some point, Indigenous people came to feel a sense of ownership of the leprosaria. For, in spite of their close connections with the people and places of their origins, long-term patients also came to see the leprosaria as their homes. In part, this attachment was the result of patients' physical and psychological dependence on the institutions, the Sisters, and other patients, and their yearnings may have reflected more the hardships of facing independence in an often much less supportive outside world. One ex-patient from East Arm told medical superintendent John Hargrave that when he had first arrived as a child,

C. Robson, *Missionary Women, Leprosy and Indigenous Australians, 1936–1986*, https://doi.org/10.1007/978-3-031-05796-0_11

> I was a bit worried, you know, because I wanted to come back here to Elcho Island. It took me a long time to know everyone there and get to like them... And the two years went past and I wanted to stay there [East Arm]. I didn't worry for my father any more...I got used to the people over there.[1]

Some patients tried to evade discharge; others, such as some Fantome Island patients discharged to Palm Island, contrived to return to the leprosarium by refusing their medication.[2] The problem was solved for a few patients who, cleared medically for discharge, stayed on or returned as members of staff. The published narrative of Jack Gibbs recounting how he and his wife, Nancy, both ex-patients, returned to East Arm reads almost as a homecoming after an itinerant interlude away from the leprosarium, with the pair effortlessly slipping back into work routines, domesticity, and the company of familiar faces.[3]

The small groups of elderly and debilitated patients remaining on closure of the leprosaria illustrate most poignantly the roots of this attachment. Of those left at Derby in 1986, for example, four who had been admitted between forty-six and fifty years previously did not know "any other home except the leprosarium."[4] Jack Gibbs wrote that on the closure of East Arm, he and Nancy were the only ones left "because we had nowhere to go."[5] Mostly, these patients wanted to remain there for the rest of their days but governments could not justify the cost of maintaining the institutions for so few residents. High-dependence patients were moved to nursing homes or hospital wards. As Michelle Moran observed of Carville and Kalaupapa residents, if it came to a choice between a hospital ward and the settlement-styled leprosarium, Australian patients preferred the latter where there was at least some space and natural surroundings.[6]

Feelings of attachment by patients to the leprosaria were also premised on their importance as places where formative and often extraordinary experiences had jointly occurred. Children developed into adults, forged relationships, and became parents. But they also forsook their newborns and regularly fare-welled their dying friends; they adjusted to a different way of life, and confronted severe illness, the probability of disfigurement and disability, and the prospect of early death. Patient communities at best were sources of mutual support against the suffering, loneliness and indignity of forced isolation, the strong helping the frail, the mature protecting and guiding the young.[7] These shared distinctive experiences were the nexus of emergent collective identities among the patients and their offspring, defined by association with each particular leprosarium, and surviving decades after these institutions closed.

Oral history testimonials suggest that strong interpersonal connections were also formed between some long-term patients and the Sisters and that, to some extent, the latter also identified with the patient group. Sr Camille of Derby leprosarium explained, "we realised the terrible emotional trauma they went through. We had a tremendous bond."[8] As Katharine Massam has written of a comparable situation at New Norcia Mission, it seems difficult to reconcile this claim to the same emotional space as the patients with the missionaries' role in upholding compulsory detention, the main cause of such "trauma."[9] But, like the Indigenous mission residents of whom Massam writes, leprosarium patients did not necessarily align their religious carers with the government policies that saw their removal from their families. Some, instead, identified with the women, seeing them also as dislocated from family life and distant homes. They highlighted their constancy and care, sometimes contrasting them to what they felt was desertion and coldness by government officers.[10] A patient from Derby leprosarium said that "they are like my own sisters" and when one died, he wrote, that she "looked after me for so long, it is hard to believe she won't be around."[11] Sandy Boyd, a patient who spent many years at Fantome Island, described the Sisters as "better than your own family."[12] So, in some cases, restrictive state policies, rather than divide Sisters and patients, served to meld them together, to form, in Massam's words, "a family of outsiders."[13]

Some ex-patients' memories indicate that, as child patients, their relations with the Sisters had been fractious but, with the passage of time and changes to life circumstances, their perspectives of the women had softened. One man remembered that "Sr Benedicta was the toughest when we do wrong things, like smokes and so on. We were bad—we knew we were bad at East Arm."[14] With a hindsight reminiscent of past pupils of many a strict schoolteacher, some patients expressed gratitude for this uncompromising approach. One ex-patient of Derby recalled when he used to "get stubborn for small things and neglect my dressings and there she was, Sr Francis, as stern as she was, giving me orders."[15] Philomena, a Northern Territory ex-patient, was grateful that she had a strict upbringing with the Sisters, contrasting it with what she considered the lax attitude of the younger people in her community to work. The

Sisters "taught me right from wrong. That's the good thing about them missionaries, I suppose. They tell you to do this and that."[16]

For many of the Sisters, particularly those of the Sisters of St John of God (SSJG) and the Franciscan Missionaries of Mary (FMM) who, individually, had very long associations with the work, the leprosaria, and the patients were core to their lives. As with the patients, some had hardly known a life other than this one. Mother Alphonsus SJG and Mother Peter OLHC (later Sister Kenan FMM), aged in their seventies, were still on duty at Derby and Fantome Island respectively in the 1970s, the latter having left for a brief time in the 1940s to enter the FMM congregation so that she could continue her work. Other Sisters who could not remain onsite lived for much of their retirement within the communities of their former patients, at Derby or Palm Island, for example.

In appeals to the government in 1969 and 1970 to keep the leprosarium open rather than sending the last patients to Palm Island Hospital, the Fantome Islander Superior evinced concern for the future of both the remaining patients and the Sisters. "I think it would be too bad to take away their freedom on this beautiful Island."[17] She then adopted the same rationale as that of the SSJG Sisters forty years earlier when they were requesting the Channel Island nursing work. "Above all for the spiritual good of such patients so much could be done… We should be sorry to see these poor patients go back to drink themselves to death or to be more or less outcasts among the people."[18] Again, Indigenous patients were depicted as prone to moral decline and abandonment without the Sisters' influence and support. And, again, there was a sense that, however devastating the separation of one group from the other would be to the patients, it would be at least equally so to the Sisters themselves.

It was not only the link to the individual patients that was important, especially to younger Sisters who had to consider their future positions in the event of the closure of the leprosaria. Sr Camille decided to leave Derby leprosarium when she knew it was going to close. "I didn't want to be caught out. In 1974, I did child and maternal health in the eastern states then went to Pilbura, then to Balgo, then to Derby where I was a public health nurse for West Kimberley."[19] As it turned out, several leprosarium Sisters were able to continue to use their professional skills to some extent. Two of the Derby Sisters continued to work in public health at the new Kimberley Disease Control Unit. [20] East Arm Sisters joined the Northern Territory's new centre for leprosy control at Katherine in the role of educators of Indigenous health workers and lay nurses.[21] Those from Fantome Island young enough to continue working were posted to Mt Isa to take up pastoral work. Yet, for these women, leprosarium work was never an ordinary job to be replaced easily by another when the institutions closed. We are reminded of that deep connection they found between the day-to-day nursing and their spirituality by the words of Sr Antoinette from Derby leprosarium, middle-aged in 1978. She perhaps spoke for many of her generation of leprosarium Sisters when she confided to another Sister, "I realise that the work is not the 'be all and end all' of everything—but combined with the apostolic activity—no doubt, it leads us all closer to the Lord."[22]

Former patients, Sisters, and doctors have found it important to commemorate their leprosarium experiences. On special occasions, groups have gathered at their respective sites—now dry and silent places—to exchange stories, mourn those in the graves, and pick their way through the crumbling remnants of their past. Sadly, due to government sanitation practices, most buildings have been destroyed, except for at Derby, the last to close. Three of the four leprosarium sites in this study—Channel and Fantome Islands and Derby—have been granted government heritage status, officially acknowledging the vital roles they continue to play in attesting to past Indigenous health policies and as places of community belonging and shared memories of former staff and of patients and their families.[23]

But to divert one's gaze from these repositories of memory to the people themselves is to realise that death, loss, and sorrow are not the only legacies of the Indigenous leprosarium system. And that Raphael Cilento's chilling pronouncement in the 1930s that Indigenous leprosarium patients, once detained, should never return to their home communities was not sustained. Not only did hundreds of people survive to live long lives outside the leprosarium, but they picked up the threads to take their places once again in society as family and community members. Many went on to become powerful and inspirational figures in their own communities and in the wider fields of Indigenous culture, health, religion, and in Indigenous rights movements. Some who have appeared in the public record may be mentioned here: Uniting Church minister, artist, land rights activist, and community elder, Dr Gawirrin Gumana of north-east Arnhem Land; health worker, Molly Wardaguga of Maningrida; senior Kimberley lawman David Mowaljarlai; Turkey Creek artists, Timmy Timms, Paddy Bedford, and Winnie Budburria, also a community Catholic religious leader; and Queensland elder, Selwyn Eggmolesse.[24]

What seems to have set these people apart is perhaps best articulated by Dr Gumana who attributes his world perspective partly to many years spent at Channel Island and then at East Arm: "I have three angles now on life and I try to make them agree with one another: the Yolngu, the Western and then there is God's, above all, looking down …I was still a warrior but not with spears, no, with my speech and tongue."[25] Ex-patients have been effective leaders because they have been able to gain some understanding of both Western and Indigenous world views and they are adept at operating in both spheres. These people never lost their longing for their land. They were able, to a large extent, to maintain their spiritual links while in the leprosaria by painting, singing, dancing, and speaking language. At the same time, particularly the young patients, saw their worlds broaden as they shared lives with others from different backgrounds and became familiarised with diverse cultures, languages, and religious/spiritual beliefs. Education in English, Christianity and Western ways by the Sisters empowered Indigenous patients in their later interactions with white Australians at various levels. Specific skills learnt in the leprosarium have been seen by patients as beneficial in their own personal survival and development as well as in assisting others in their communities.

There is perhaps some mitigating irony in the idea that institutions defined by their austerity and oppression of freedom have played host to lively exchanges of cultural practices and religious beliefs. It suggests that the patients did not accept wholesale the single cultural and religious model promoted by the Catholic missionaries; they exercised choice as they incorporated those aspects that worked for them into their own systems of belief. Testimonies of some ex-patients suggest that the Judaic-Christian scriptures offered an explanation of, and sometimes an antidote to, the depredation and disease inflicted upon them by colonialism. Noel Loos has put it this way: "Aboriginal Christians had experienced the crucifixion of colonisation and contempt. Now it seemed that as a people they would experience the triumph over suffering of the resurrection."[26] His observation aligns closely to accounts given by Gija people Paddy Bedford and Winnie Budburria of the Eastern Kimberley, both of whom first encountered Christianity in the Derby leprosarium. For Bedford, the persecution of Christ by Roman soldiers paralleled atrocities visited on family members and friends by European settlers in the Kimberley:

> When we got to know the story of Jesus we said 'That's Our Story.' We were like Jesus-he was killed too... We were crying for our people who were killed. That's why we can like Mary and Jesus. They are like us Aboriginal people.[27]

Budburria saw Christianity as a healing force, enabling her to "get really better for going back to our home country."[28] After only a few years in the leprosarium, she was discharged and became an enthusiastic catechist, drawing a following known as the "Catholic mob" at Turkey Creek and, in the 1960s, at Kununurra. As typifies many Indigenous interpretations of Christianity, Budburria's Catholicism was fused with Indigenous spirituality.[29] Budburria indicates that it was readily accommodated by the pastoral station people whose connections with "the other old way" had dissipated after many of the old people had been removed to government reserves decades previously.[30] For Budburria, this form of Christianity represented a vital spiritual reinvigoration for a community beleaguered by loss, violence, and disease.

Conclusions

The main aim of this book has been to lay bare the collaboration by government and church authorities to manage Indigenous people with leprosy in Australia. Documents from state and missionary archives have provided ample evidence of policies and practices of racially targeted oppression tempered with nursing and medical treatment, general care and support, and advocacy of rights, provided mainly by the Catholic Sisters but also by doctors, lay staff, and other missionaries. I have argued that this approach was based on Christian tradition, concurrent international medical knowledge and models of leprosy policy, and the entry of Catholic women religious into leprosarium nursing in the colonised world. But it was also driven by local forces. Coinciding with the White Australia Policy, leprosy policy privileged the health of white Australians in the northern frontiers over Indigenous Australians and aligned with 'protection,' and to some degree, after the Second World War, assimilationist principles. It was underpinned by medico-bureaucratic preconceptions of the Indigenous as irresponsible and uncivilised, and justified by the dearth of health and medical services in remote communities. Yet, the promises of high standard treatment and conditions in the institutions were seldom fulfilled, either because of the inherent difficulties of their remote locations or government parsimony. The efforts of staff and patients often had to substitute for inadequate provisions and care. The expected benefits of the therapeutic advances of the 1950s and 1960s bypassed many patients, depriving them of their freedom, independence, and return to their families and homes.

The nature of leprosarium isolation for the Indigenous was partially determined by the expansion of the Australian Catholic mission enterprise in northern Australia from the interwar period, which facilitated the involvement of Catholic Sister nurses in leprosy caregiving. I have argued here that the individual women, propelled by their strong Christian faith, incorporated their culture, values, and particular ways of caregiving into the leprosaria, seeking to assuage the dire effects of removal and incarceration.

In many respects, this is a story of ideals rather than realities. We learn of what authorities, both religious and secular, wanted, and perhaps expected, of Indigenous patients as they entered the leprosarium and were ushered into work teams, classes, chapels, and clinics. And it tells us of the aspirations of the Europeans who put these systems in place: for the Sisters, God's grace; for the doctors, medical achievement and for the health bureaucrat, the containment of disease; for many of them, the sincere hope for improved health and welfare of the patients.

But the other side of this history is the reality for the people most affected, the Indigenous. Testimonies by former patients and some government correspondence have shown that patients, when their health permitted, did not passively accept the projects and plans of their European overseers. They either actively engaged with them, negotiated them, as for example with wages for labour, or resisted them. They strove to keep links with family, culture, and country alive, while forming new relationships, making new families, and embracing multiple cultures, beliefs, and languages. Notwithstanding the enormity of death and suffering, this history is also about the overcoming of oppression and disease. As much as it's about what Europeans wanted for them, it's about the lives Indigenous people made for themselves and each other in the institutions.

Notes

1. "Yawirongga" (fictitious name) quoted in Cawte, John. 2001. *Healers of Arnhem Land*. Marleston: J.B. Books, 63.

2. Ex-patient (name confidential) to Secretary, Relatives and Friends Association, 7 October 1954. (Director of Native Affairs Office, 3A/153, Correspondence, Aboriginal and Torres Strait Islander, ITM505017), Queensland State Archives (QSA).
3. Gibbs, Jack.1995. *Son of Jimmy*. Darwin: Historical Society of the Northern Territory, 113, 118, 121.
4. 'Derby Leprosarium (report on future of leprosarium),' October 1985, 2. (Health Department, LEP-01v1, Cons 4956), State Records Office Western Australia.
5. Gibbs, *Son of Jimmy*, 121.
6. Moran, Michelle T. 2007. *Colonising Leprosy: Imperialism and the Politics of Public Health in the United States*. Chapel Hill: University of North Carolina Press, 198–200.
7. For example, Laurelle D'Antoine said that when her young son was taken to Derby Leprosarium, "The Aboriginal people out there were very very good to him...He started to get used to the people and I've got a lot of time for them. People ... used to take him fishing and camping so he wouldn't have time to think about his illness and family" (Wright, Edie. 2001. *Full Circle: From Mission to Community—A Family Story*. Fremantle: Fremantle Arts Centre Press. 209–210).
8. Poidevin, Sister Camille SJG. Interview with author. Typed transcript. Recorded at Derby, Western Australia, November 17, 2008.
9. Massam, Katherine. 2008. '"That there was love in this home": The Benedictine Missionary Sisters at New Norcia,' In *Evangelists of Empire? Missionaries in Colonial History*, ed. Amanda Barry, Joanna Cruickshank, Andrew Brown-May and Patricia Grimshaw. Melbourne: School of Historical Studies, The University of Melbourne, 202.
10. "Mary" (former patient, Fantome Island Leprosarium), interviewer unknown, n.d. Sound recording. (North Queensland Oral History Project, JCU ID 521, Parts 1 & 2), James Cook University; Pan, Eileen. 1997. 'Pray for Us.' In *The Telling of Stories: A Spiritual Journey of Kimberley Aboriginal People*, ed. Peter Bibby. Western Australia: Catholic Education Office, Kimberley Region, 58–59.
11. Former patient and family (names confidential), 'In Memory of Sr Francis Dunne' (2.42Y), Sisters of St John of God Archives Broome (SSJGB).
12. Boyd, Sandy. 198–? Interview with Siobhan McHugh, Siobhan McHugh Collection of Australian Social History. Sound recording (ORAL TRC 2761/5), National Library of Australia.
13. Massam, 'That there was love in this home,' 202.
14. Yawirongga quoted in Cawte, *Healers of Arnhem Land*, 63.
15. Former patient and family, 'In Memory of Sr Francis Dunne.'

16. Kerinaiua, Philomena. C. 2002. 'Philomena's Story.' In *So Far From Home: Oral Histories of the Stolen Generations*, ed. Lana Quall. Katherine: Diwurruwurru-jaru Aboriginal Corporation, 30.
17. Bellemare, Sr Ubald to Killoran, Patrick (Director, Queensland Department of Aboriginal and Islander Affairs), September 7, 1969. (Director of Native Affairs Office, 3A/157, Correspondence, Aboriginal and Torres Strait Islander, ID ITM505023), QSA.
18. Sr Ubald to Killoran, August 25, 1970. (3A/157, ITM505023), QSA.
19. Poidevin, Sr Camille, Interview with author.
20. Murray, Sally. 2002. *We Never Counted Hours: A Brief History of the Kimberley Disease Control Unit, 3–4*. Derby: privately published, SSJGB.
21. Leahy, Sr Kathleen. 1982. 'After'39 Years'—Farewell to East Arm,' *The Annals* of *Our Lady of the Sacred Heart*, 6.
22. Kelly, Sr Antoinette to Sr Stella, October 7, 1978. (2.4 K) SSJGB.
23. Channel Island: Commonwealth Government Heritage Register Place ID 14,869, May 14, 1991; Derby: Western Australia State Heritage Register Place No. 02980; Fantome Island: Queensland State Heritage Register Place ID 602,798, June 8, 2012.
24. Rothwell, Nicolas. 2007. *Another Country*. Melbourne: Black Inc., 11–19; Kildea, Sue. 2005. 'Molly Wardagga.' In *Aboriginal and Islander Health Worker Journal* 30 (6), 3–5; *Visions of Mowanjum: Aboriginal Writings from the Kimberley*, Adelaide: Rigby, 1980, 97–99; Dolk, Michiel. 2007. 'Are we Strangers in this place?' In *Paddy Bedford*, ed. Paddy Bedford with Russell Storer. Sydney: Museum of Contemporary Art, 17–19; *From Digging Sticks to Writing Sticks: Stories of Kija Women as told to Veronica Ryan, Eileen Bray & Mary Thomas (trans.)*, Leederville: Catholic Education Office of Western Australia, 2001, 146–153.
25. Gawirrin Gumana quoted in Rothwell, *Another Country*, 13.
26. Loos, Noel. 2007. *White Christ, Black Cross: The Emergence of a Black Church*. Canberra: Aboriginal Studies Press, 15.
27. Bedford, 'God Knows,' in Bibby, *The Telling of Stories*, 37. Killings of Indigenous people at Bedford Downs and Mistake Creek in the first half of the twentieth century have been revisited in the stories and art of Eastern Kimberley people, such as Winnie Budburria, Paddy Bedford, and Timmy Timms. See Smith, Pam. 2007. 'Conflict: Ways of Remembering.' *Journal of Australian Studies* 91, 9–23; Langton, Marcia. 'Goowoomji's World.' In Bedford, *Paddy Bedford*, 55.
28. Winnie Budburria quoted in *From Digging Sticks to Writing Sticks*, 49.

29. Shaw, Kevin. 2003. *Mates: Images and Stories from the Kimberley.* Melbourne: Australian Scholarly Publishing, 4. N.B. The extent and nature of such syncretism cannot be ascertained here. As Noel McMaster has argued, "A critical and thorough assessment of the [Catholic] church's cross-cultural evangelising among Indigenous people of the Kimberley is yet to be seriously undertaken" (McMaster, Noel. 2008. *The Catholic Church in Jaru and Gija Country.* Melbourne: David Lovell Publishing, 209).
30. Winnie Budburria quoted in *From Digging Sticks to Writing Sticks*, 151–153.

Terminology

Note regarding the names of the leprosaria:

Local Indigenous people have names for the leprosaria or their locations:

> Derby leprosarium—*Bungarun*
> Channel Island leprosarium—*Quarantine* (with various other spellings)
> Fantome Island—*Eumilli*

To avoid confusion, this book follows the convention used in historic documents, and refers to these places by their European names.

Leprosy

The term 'leprosy' was replaced by 'Hansen's disease' in common usage after the middle of the twentieth century due to the associated stigma of the former term. Because this book is situated in the historical periods before and after this change, the term 'leprosy' is used.

Leprosarium

Institution for detainment and treatment of people diagnosed with leprosy.

C. Robson, *Missionary Women, Leprosy and Indigenous Australians, 1936–1986*, https://doi.org/10.1007/978-3-031-05796-0

Lazaret

Two meanings: 1. leprosarium; 2. site set aside for detainment of people identified as having leprosy.

Indigenous

With first letter capitalised, describes person of Australian Aborigines and Torres Strait Islander descent; with lower-case first letter, describes any other First Nations person.

Mixed Descent/Mixed Race

Describes person with Indigenous heritage plus another ethnicity. It is necessary only to make this distinction as it was relevant historically. Historical documents distinguish between people with parents who were both Indigenous ('full-bloods'); those who had one Indigenous parent ('half-castes'); and those who had one Indigenous grand-parent ('quarter-caste' or 'quadroon').

White/European

Used interchangeably to describe Australians of European or Anglo-Celtic background.

Aboriginal/Aborigine

In historic documents. Refers to people of Indigenous Australian and/or Torres Strait Islander descent.

Abbreviations

BELRA: British Empire Leprosy Relief Association
DOLSH: Daughters of Our Lady of the Sacred Heart
DNA: Department of Native Affairs
DSS: Department of Social Services
FHC: Federal Health Council
FMM: Franciscan Missionaries of Mary
MSC: Missionaries of the Sacred Heart
NHMRC: National Health and Medical Research Council
OFM: Orders of the Friars Minor
OLHC: Our Lady Help of Christians
RFA: Relatives and Friends Association
SAC: Society of the Catholic Apostolate (Pallottines).
SSJG: Sisters of St John of God
UAM: United Aborigines Mission
UN: United Nations
WHO: World Health Organisation

C. Robson, *Missionary Women, Leprosy and Indigenous Australians, 1936–1986*, https://doi.org/10.1007/978-3-031-05796-0

Name Index

C. Robson, *Missionary Women, Leprosy and Indigenous Australians, 1936–1986*, https://doi.org/10.1007/978-3-031-05796-0

I

J

K

L

M

Subject Index

C. Robson, *Missionary Women, Leprosy and Indigenous Australians, 1936–1986*, https://doi.org/10.1007/978-3-031-05796-0

Printed by Printforce, United Kingdom